DESIGN

MEASURE

ASSESS

IMPROVE

PERFORMANCE IMPROVEMENT in Ambulatory Care

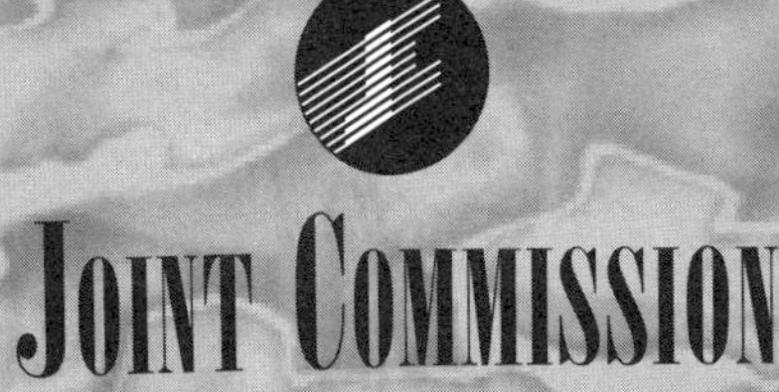

Joint Commission Mission

The mission of the Joint Commission on Accreditation of Healthcare Organizations is to improve the quality of care provided to the public through the provision of health care accreditation and related services that support performance improvement.

Joint Commission educational programs and publications support, but are separate from, the accreditation activities of the Joint Commission. Attendees at Joint Commission educational programs and purchasers of Joint Commission publications receive no special consideration or treatment in, or confidential information about, the accreditation process.

Printed in the U.S.A. 5 4 3 2 1

Requests for permission to reprint or make copies of any part of this work should be mailed to:

Permissions Editor
Department of Publications
Joint Commission on Accreditation of Healthcare Organizations
One Renaissance Boulevard
Oakbrook Terrace, IL 60181
http://www.jcaho.org

ISBN: 0-86688-528-5

Library of Congress Catalog Number: 96-079557

Contents

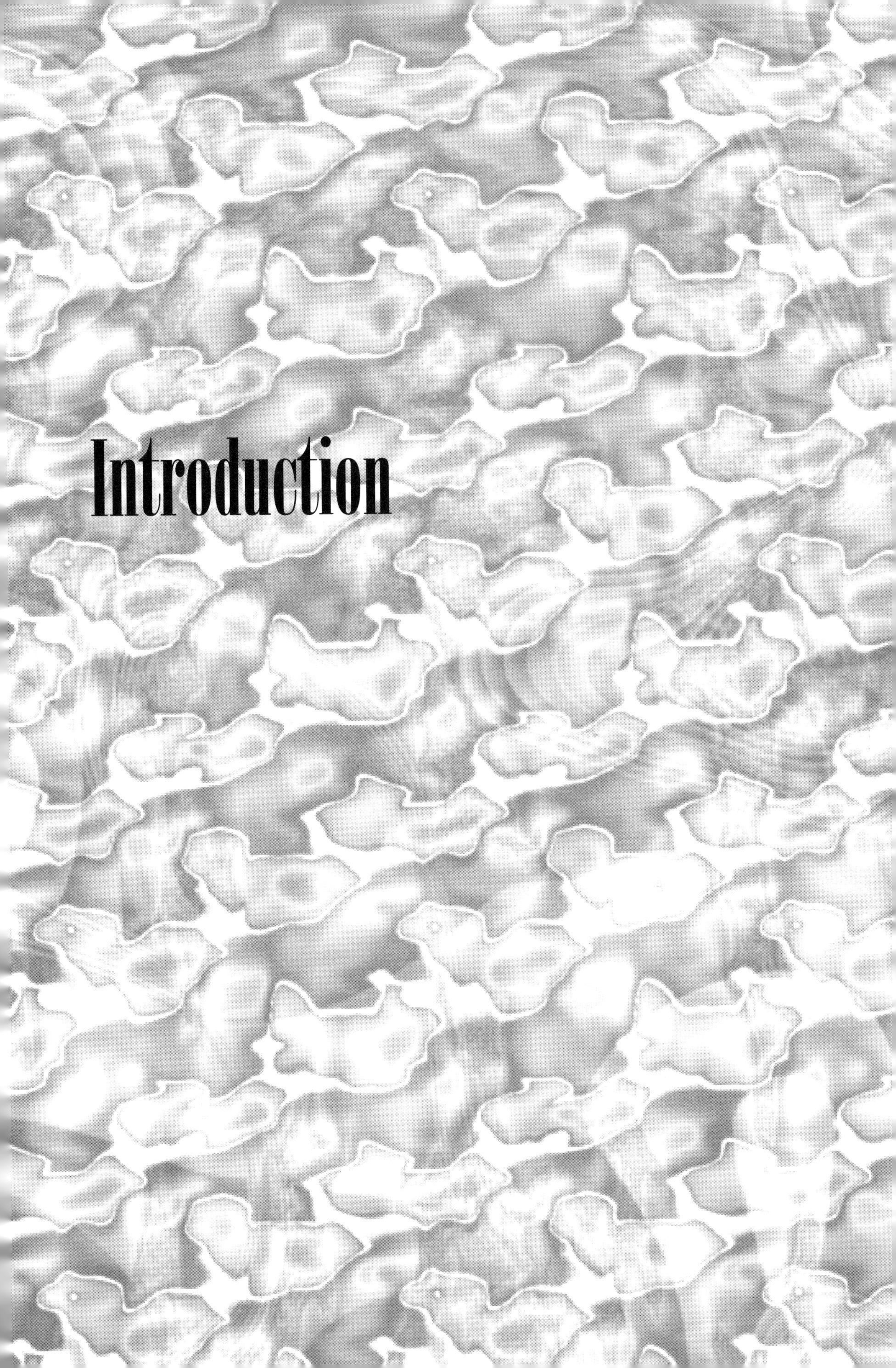

Introduction

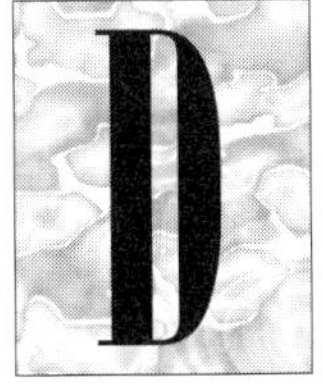

riven by its mission, "to improve the quality of care provided to the public through the provision of health care accreditation and related services that support performance improvement," the Joint Commission has incorporated contemporary knowledge about organization excellence into its quality improvement approach or framework. This approach is designed to help health care organizations achieve high-quality care, optimal outcomes, and efficient use of resources.

Providing high quality care is challenging—it means that treatment is efficacious and appropriate, available when needed, and delivered in a timely fashion. Equally important, care must be provided in a respectful and caring manner. It must also be effective, safe, efficient, and well coordinated over time and among practitioners and settings.

Ambulatory health care organizations* that systematically improve the quality of care delivery can expect superior care outcomes, more competitive costs, and high levels of client satisfaction. Delivery of high-quality care is directly related to performance of critical organizational systems, and the effective, coordinated performance of multiple jobs and tasks.

In developing a quality improvement framework, the Joint Commission carefully synthesized a wide range of available theories, methods, and tools, and added its own experience. This approach gives professionals the methods they need to systematically and scientifically enhance care processes and their outcomes. The framework has grown out of the long-standing search for quality and the efforts of literally hundreds of health care organizations and professionals.

The framework is compatible with total quality management and continuous quality improvement strategies. These strategies stress the importance of leadership, and understanding external and internal customer needs. They also

---

*When the term *ambulatory care* is used, it includes surgery centers, birthing centers, cardiac catheterization units, chiropractic clinics, community health services, corporate health services, correctional facilities, dental centers, dialysis centers, endoscopy centers, group practices/primary care centers, imaging centers, independent practitioner practices, infusion therapy lithotripsy units, migrant health services, military and veterans affairs clinics, mobile speciality units, oncology centers, ophthalmology surgery centers, oral and maxillofacial centers, podiatric centers, public health departments, radiation and MRI centers, recovery care centers, research centers, rehabilitation centers, rural health centers, student health services, urgent and emergency care centers, women's health centers, and Native American health centers.

include opportunities for outcomes-driven design of new products and services, broad use of measurement systems, data-driven performance assessment, and systematic design and redesign of important organization processes and functions.

The primary goals of the Joint Commission's framework are to

- emphasize the link between an organization's performance of important functions and its care outcomes, the costs to achieve these outcomes and judgments about the quality and value of its services;
- illustrate how an organization can mesh the rich variety of concepts, methods, and strategies independently developed over the past several decades with an operational performance improvement system relevant to health care; and
- demonstrate that the effectiveness with which an organization manages its relationship with the external environment is as important to the fulfillment of its mission as the effectiveness with which it manages its internal environment.

This book describes the Joint Commission's performance improvement standards application to ambulatory care organizations. Initially, it provides an overview of the principles and history on which the framework is built and introduces the primary components of the framework, which include the

- external environment, including the political, social, economic, and other societal forces that influence how an ambulatory care organization delivers service and fulfills its mission;
- internal environment, particularly the governance, management, clinical, and support activities that affect care delivery and outcome; and
- cycle for improving performance, which is a practical method for improving processes.

Subsequent chapters explore each stage of the improvement cycle and present examples adapted from the experiences of different types of ambulatory health care facilities, both large and small, independent and hospital based. Each chapter contains numerous examples from a variety of settings, including surgery centers; women's health centers; ambulatory components of hospitals, integrated delivery systems, and HMOs; radiology centers; endoscopy centers; correctional facilities; student health services; community health centers; and veterans affairs medical centers. Appendix A is an excerpt from the *National Library of Healthcare*

Indicators: Health Plan and Network Edition. Appendix B offers some suggestions on how to promote effective teamwork.

This book is a practical and pragmatic guide. It can be used to acquire an overview of performance improvement concepts and methods. It can also be used as a reference tool and resource for organizations to help carry out their improvement activities.

Summary

This improvement framework presents many challenges to health care organizations, particularly in ambulatory health care, including redesigning care processes, promoting collaborative teamwork, systematically measuring and assessing performance, and encouraging risk taking and experimentation. The ability to proactively and effectively manage quality is perhaps the only way that organizations will prosper in the face of stringent resource constraints and increasing demands for better care and service outcomes.

Reference

National Library of Healthcare Indicators: Health Plan and Network Edition. Oakbrook Terrace, IL: Joint Commission on Accreditation of Healthcare Organizations, 1997.

CHAPTER 1: Overview

Chapter Highlights

Underlying Principles

- The purpose of ambulatory care is to maximize a patient's health and to use resources efficiently and appropriately.
- Care outcomes and use of resources are affected by the nine measurable dimensions of performance: efficacy, appropriateness, availability, timeliness, effectiveness, continuity, safety, efficiency, and respect and caring.
- The degree to which ambulatory care organizations fulfill these nine dimensions of performance is strongly influenced by the design and operation of a series of important functions and processes.
- Leadership and collaboration are essential for ambulatory health care professionals, especially in the current health care environment.
- An organization's performance is evident by measuring patient outcomes,

Continued on page 8.

Continued from page 7.

customer satisfaction and perception of quality, and costs.

Components of the Framework for Improving Performance

The framework incorporates the best ideas and methods into a flexible approach to improvement. The three basic components of the framework are the

- external environment;
- internal environment; and
- cycle for improving performance.

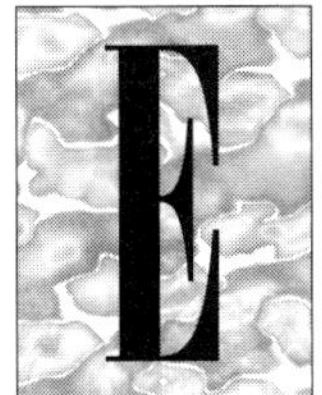

xtraordinary forces are at work reshaping health care today in the United States. Everywhere we look—newspapers, television news broadcasts, magazines, health care publications—commentaries highlight the intense concern about the future of health care. Key issues include the availability, quality, and value of health care.

These concerns are shared not only by the recipients of care, but also by care providers, the public, purchasers, payers, accreditors, and regulators. Together, these concerns are fueling unprecedented efforts to understand and improve how health care is delivered.

In the past decade, cost-containment strategies, including prospective payment plans, capitation, and managed care, have dramatically reshaped the delivery of health care services. The emerging trends in health care delivery have included

- movement from hospital-based toward community-based care;
- movement from inpatient to outpatient care;
- expansion of gatekeeping functions and case management services for cost containment and to further integrate care;
- design of shared risk and collaborative reimbursement models;
- adoption of outcomes research and disease management concepts; and
- greater emphasis on health promotion and wellness.

It is in this context that ambulatory services now stand, facing increasing scrutiny and oversight. Performance data are vital now, when policy makers, payers, and patients and their families are demanding that organizations provide information to demonstrate the value of their services.

Therefore, the missions of the Joint Commission and the ambulatory care organization seeking accreditation are strongly aligned. Both are driven to improve the quality of care provided to the public. Since the inception of its ambulatory accreditation program, the Joint Commission has carried out this mission through several ongoing activities:

- Developing and gaining national consensus on standards for ambulatory care;
- Evaluating organizations to determine compliance with the standards;
- Educating and leading efforts in performance improvement and other issues central to quality; and

- Developing process and outcome indicators useful both to organizations and to the Joint Commission in evaluating the level of performance of important functions.

Underlying Principles

One product of the Joint Commission's activities is a framework for improving performance. This framework rests on several related, interlocking principles. These principles focus on the purpose of health care, how health care is delivered, and how health care is improved. These principles are briefly reviewed here. In the remaining chapters of this book, these principles will be demonstrated in examples and discussion.

The Purpose of Health Care

The central purpose of health care is to maximize the health and comfort of the people served and provide the highest quality care in a cost-effective manner, regardless of the specific setting or service. Many variables (from both the external and internal environments) influence the success of an organization in achieving this central purpose. For example, competence of the clinicians who provide care, the availability of adequate staffing, and the patient's or family's ability to participate in their own care all affect outcomes.

Ambulatory care organizations also face a unique challenge. Ambulatory outcomes are difficult to develop and assess, perhaps by virtue of their broad treatment perspective and the extent to which care is influenced by social, environmental, and medical factors. The work of ambulatory care organizations also spans a huge array of services (such as, preventive care, intravenous therapy, outpatient surgery and diagnostic tests, rehabilitation) and care settings (such as, primary care clinic, surgery center, endoscopy center), which adds to the complexity.

Specific challenges relevant to ambulatory care organizations include

- the tracking of patients receiving multiple service from multiple practitioners in multiple settings;
- sophisticated information management systems need to be built, enabling organizations to identify relationships between care, cost, and care outcomes;
- maintaining continuity of care is a problem in some ambulatory care settings, such as correctional health facilities and student health clinics.

These organizations often have difficulty obtaining health information on patients from hospitals, specialists, and other entities.
- many important, high-volume clinical activities are difficult to quantify and measure; and
- many factors in addition to treatment may influence the course of clinical activities (for example, patient life-style, patient/family compliance with treatment).

To meet this challenge, ambulatory care organizations must improve quality and service outcomes, use resources efficiently, and satisfy internal/external customers. This framework is designed to help organizations pursue the goal of achieving optimal care outcomes at the lowest possible cost, using the appropriate level and amount of service.

Nine Dimensions of Performance

Nine important dimensions of ambulatory care organization performance affect the quality of outcomes and resource use. The dimensions are divided into two groups that comprise a traditional definition of quality: 1) Was the right thing done? and 2) Was it done right? One advantage of using the dimensions of performance is that they can be measured and improved, allowing an organization to track its progress. The nine dimensions of performance are efficacy, appropriateness, availability, timeliness, effectiveness, continuity, safety, efficiency, and respect and caring. The dimensions are defined in Table 1-1, page 12.

Functions and Processes

The degree to which care fulfills the nine dimensions of performance is strongly influenced by the design and operation of a series of important clinical and organization functions. These functions include direct care activities (such as assessment, treatment, and education), as well as governance, management, and support services (such as information management and human resources management).

A *function* is defined as a group of processes with a common goal. A *process* is defined as a series of linked, goal-directed activities. For example, information management could be viewed as a function and data entry as a process within that function. Similarly, medication use could be viewed as a function and medication administration and clinical monitoring as processes within that function.

Table 1-1. Nine Dimensions of Performance

Doing the Right Thing

The **efficacy** of the procedure or treatment in relation to the patient's condition.

The degree to which the care of the patient has been shown to accomplish the desired or projected outcome(s).

The **appropriateness** of a specific test, procedure, or service to meet the patient's needs.

The degree to which the care provided is relevant to the patient's clinical needs, given the current state of knowledge.

Doing the Right Thing Well

The **availability** of a needed test, procedure, treatment, or service to the patient who needs it.

The degree to which appropriate care is available to meet the patient's needs.

The **timeliness** with which a needed test, procedure, treatment, or service is provided to the patient.

The degree to which care is provided to the patient at the most beneficial or necessary time.

The **effectiveness** with which tests, procedures, treatments, and services are provided.

The degree to which the care is provided in the correct manner, given the current state of knowledge, to achieve the desired or projected outcome(s) for the patient.

The **continuity** of the services provided to the patient with respect to other services, practitioners, and providers, and over time.

The degree to which the care for the patient is coordinated among practitioners, among organizations, and over time.

The **safety** of the patient (and others) to whom the services are provided.

The degree to which the risk of an intervention and the risk in the care environment are reduced for the patient and others, including the health care provider.

The **efficiency** with which services are provided.

The relationship between the outcomes (results of care) and the resources used to deliver patient care.

The **respect and caring** with which services are provided.

The degree to which the patient or a designee is involved in his or her own care decisions and to which those providing services do so with sensitivity and respect for the patient's needs, expectations, and individual differences.

The processes involved in providing care and services to patients are never isolated tasks, but rather a series of activities that form important functions. The framework uses this important idea and focuses on the design, measurement, assessment, and improvement of functions as well as of the processes within them. The framework is not limited to improvement of direct care functions, but clearly recognizes that governance, management, and support functions also significantly influence care outcomes.

Table 1-2. Important Functions

Patient-focused Functions	Organization Functions
■ Patient Rights and Organization Ethics	■ Improving Organization Performance
■ Assessment of Patient	■ Leadership
■ Care of Patient	■ Management of the Environment of Care
■ Education of Patients and Family	■ Management of Human Resources
■ Continuity of Care	■ Management of Information
	■ Surveillance, Prevention, and Control of Infection

The Joint Commission's standards* are divided into two major sections: patient-focused functions, which primarily involve direct and indirect care to the patient, and organization functions, which do not involve direct care to the individual (see Table 1-2, above). This focus on improving organization performance through attention to processes and functions has several important implications described in this book, including the following:

Effective care must cross organization boundaries. In ambulatory care organizations, patient care is provided by teams of interdependent staff, whose individual efforts must be well coordinated to achieve common goals. These goals cannot be accomplished unless processes and communication can freely cross intraorganization boundaries; therefore, different disciplines and different levels of staff must be able to communicate and work together effectively. In any specific design or improvement effort, one discipline alone will not be able to successfully implement a process that involves several disciplines.

In many ambulatory care organizations, the concept of teamwork is inherent in the philosophy of care. Often, care in ambulatory settings is delivered using an interdisciplinary team. Members of a team may include physicians, nurses, support personnel, and volunteers. Other team members, such as a pharmacist, dietitian, physical therapist, or recreation therapist, may be added as needed to

*Refer to your most recent copy of the Joint Commission's *Comprehensive Accreditation Manual for Ambulatory Care.*

provide additional services to the individual being served. As the treatment team grows in number of members and complexity, the need for cross-discipline collaboration also grows.

Customer-supplier relationships need to be understood. All organizations have both internal customers and suppliers (for example, departments or teams within an ambulatory care setting), and external customers (for example, patients, major employers, payers, and health plans) and suppliers (for example, drug suppliers and computer software suppliers). A critical first step in improving organization performance is defining and identifying these customer-supplier relationships and their associated work processes. Once defined, these relationships must also be evaluated on a regular basis. Work is completed by enacting a series of customer-supplier relationships. Well-designed processes facilitate these transactions effectively.

Outcomes must be defined and measured. Every process, by definition, produces results. Results may be intended and desirable, intended and undesirable, unintended and desirable, or unintended and undesirable. To determine how a process is performing, an organization can measure the activities involved in the process, and also its outcomes. As noted earlier, care outcomes in ambulatory care are likely to be more difficult to define and measure. Some likely outcome dimensions include clinical status measures, physical/functional capacity, psychosocial functioning, and family and work functioning. Measuring costs and patient satisfaction should also be considered.

Variation in processes and outcomes should be analyzed. Some variation exists in all processes and, therefore, variability in outcomes is normal. Analyzing the cause(s) and relative ranges of variation helps distinguish between a special cause (nonrecurring event) and a common or systemic cause. Analyzing variation provides useful information that can be used to improve the performance of functions and processes.

Focus on improving processes rather than on individual performance. Ordinarily, designing or improving a process to achieve performance goals is best accomplished by focusing on the process, rather than on the individuals who carry it out. Both W. Edwards Deming and Joseph M. Juran, quality improvement leaders, demonstrated that the variation in outputs may be attributed to the effect of multiple causes in a system of common cause variation, rather than to individual workers. Occasionally, a lack of knowledge, skill, sound judgment, or motivation of an individual will result in undesirable performance. Most major improvement opportunities, however, are found in processes.

Outcomes, Cost, Quality, and Value

The effect of an organization's performance of important functions can influence the

- quality of care;
- cost of services;
- satisfaction of the patients served and their family members;
- outcomes and the way they were achieved; and
- judgments of important customers, including those that patients make about the quality and value of the care or service provided.

The framework described in this book focuses on improving the results of ambulatory care (including the outcomes of care) and on making better judgments about the quality and value of care.

Improving Performance

The framework for improving performance draws on the most successful approaches to improvement in health care and business, and combines these approaches into a logical and flexible cycle to carry out a wide range of improvement activities. As noted earlier, these approaches all assume that significant opportunities for improvement will be found in designing and implementing organization functions and processes, rather than in scrutinizing an individual's performance. The key to improving performance (for example, outcomes, satisfaction, quality, and value) is in systematically designing, measuring, assessing, and improving the organization's functions and processes.

Components of the Framework for Improving Performance

The framework for improving performance reflects what an organization committed to excellence must minimally address. This framework is not limited to one method of improvement, nor is it limited soley to improving performance. It recognizes that both external issues (such as health care reform and community needs) and internal issues (such as leadership and human resources) affect an ambulatory care organization's performance. Finally, it presents an adaptable cycle for designing, measuring, assessing, and improving processes and outcomes in an ambulatory care organization.

Figure 1-1, page 17, illustrates this framework's three basic components:

- External environment;
- Internal environment; and
- Cycle for improving performance.

External Environment

Factors outside an ambulatory care organization significantly affect the way the organization designs and carries out its services (see Table 1-3, page 18). Organizations must recognize how such factors in the external environment affect the organization's internal environment, priorities, and performance improvement efforts. To stay in a proactive position, organizations should continuously survey their environment, elicit feedback from customers and others, and act accordingly. Today, ambulatory care organizations must monitor and address at least the following external forces:

- ***Health care reform.*** The need to prepare for and respond to ongoing and major reconfiguration in the health care delivery and payment systems.
- ***Purchasers.*** The need to address the expectations of purchasers (for example, HMOs, POSs, PPOs, employers, Health Care Financing Administration, insurers, patients).
- ***Accrediting organizations such as the Joint Commission.*** The need to meet nationally recognized standards.
- ***Regulators.*** The need to fulfill state and federal regulatory requirements, which affect the design of many services.
- ***Accountability.*** The need to demonstrate to others (including patients, the community, and purchasers) the quality and value of the care provided.
- ***Community needs.*** The need to understand and address the needs and expectations of the community served.
- ***Special advocacy groups.*** The need to recognize and form collaborative working relationships with groups developed to advance rights and concerns of patients served.

Consumers are most interested in

- safe and effective services;
- fair access to service;

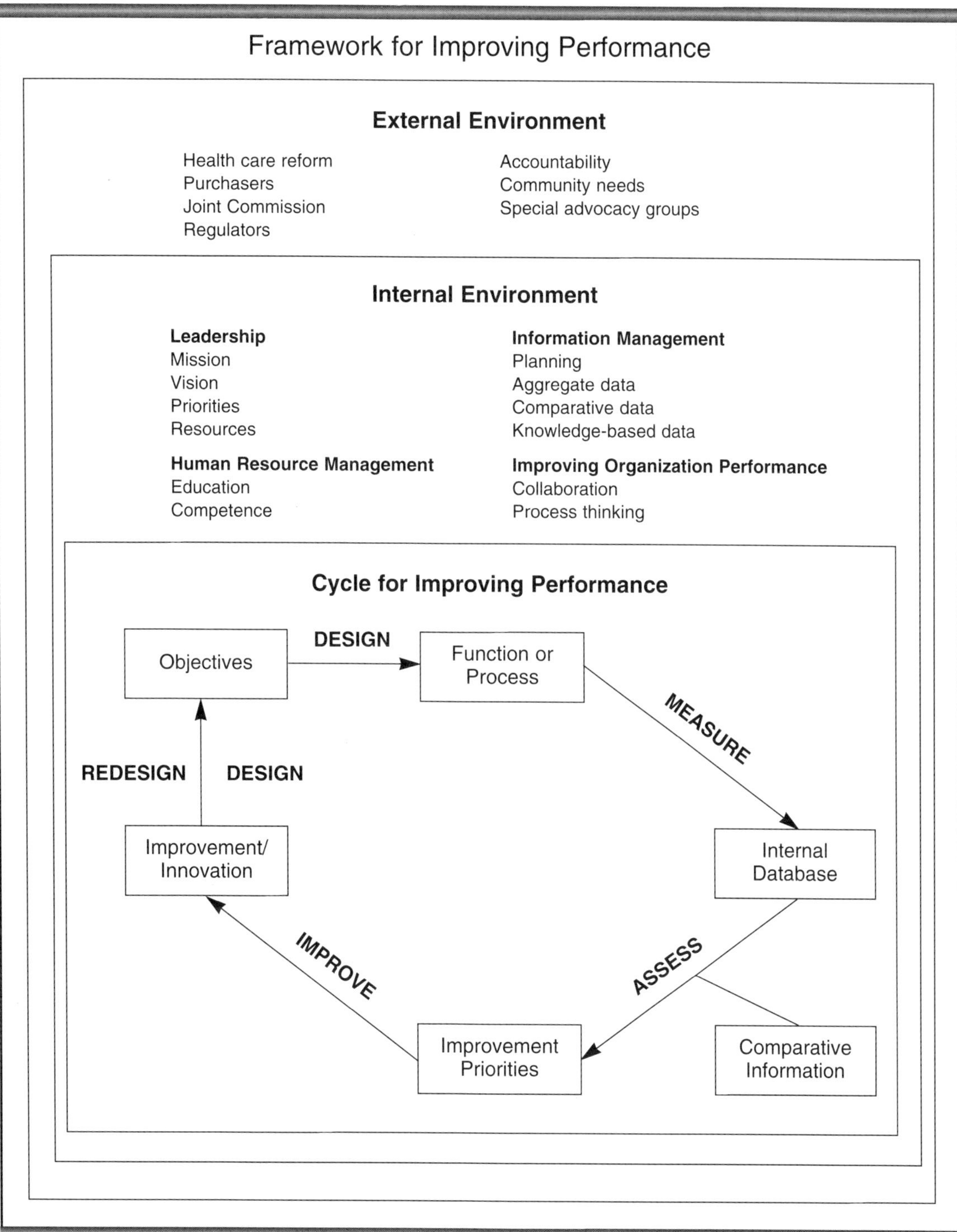

Figure 1-1. This illustration depicts the three core components of the framework for improving performance: the external environment, the internal environment, and the cycle for improving performance.

Table 1-3. Framework for Improving Performance—External Environment

External Environment	
■ Health care reform	■ Accountability
■ Purchasers	■ Community needs
■ Joint Commission	■ Special advocacy groups
■ Regulators	

- cost effectiveness; and
- the empowerment of consumers through education and board representation.

Internal Environment

The internal environment—the second component of this framework—is a blanket term for the many functions existing inside an organization that most influence performance, including efforts to design, measure, assess, and improve processes (see Table 1-4, page 19). The following internal functions are most important in determining the overall quality and value of the care and other services provided by an ambulatory care organization:

- Leadership;
- Human resources management;
- Information management; and
- Improving organization performance.

Leadership. Leaders in an ambulatory care organization typically include the members of the governing body, the chief executive officer, the clinical director, senior administrators, unit or service directors, and other senior managers. In small ambulatory care organizations, one individual may serve in more than one of these leadership roles. The internal environment is significantly shaped by the leadership of the organization. Effective leaders share certain qualities, including

- expertise in their areas of responsibility;
- knowledge about improvement, including an understanding of systems, variation, measurement, and the psychology of human behavior and motivation;

Table 1-4. Framework for Improving Performance—Internal Environment

Leadership
- Mission
- Vision
- Priorities
- Resources

Human Resources Management
- Education
- Competence

Information Management
- Planning
- Aggregate data
- Comparative data
- Knowledge-based data

Improving Organization Performance
- Collaboration
- Process thinking

- authority and willingness to allocate resources for improvement activities;
- an understanding that continuous improvement is essential to an organization's success;
- a passion for improvement;
- an understanding of organizations and of organization change; and
- vision.

One crucial responsibility for leaders is organization planning. Leaders, along with members of the organization, must define strategic plans that are consistent with the organization's mission and vision. Once developed, the leaders must then communicate these plans throughout the organization and allocate resources for their accomplishment. The Joint Commission's leadership standards require that the strategic plan set the organization's priorities for performance improvement and be aligned with the organization's mission and identified community needs. This is an enormously important activity, given the scarcity of resources and growing cost-containment forces.

Other leadership activities can also have great influence on organization performance. For example, building teamwork and fostering continuous improvement often require leaders to become better facilitators and coaches. In this role, they encourage constant learning, innovation, and risk taking. Similarly, empowerment is a concept gaining support and commitment among leaders and considered essential for successful leadership. Many effective leaders empower staff throughout the organization to acquire and apply the knowledge and skills to continuously improve processes and services. Leaders also encourage continuous improvement through their personal and direct involvement in measurement, assessment, and improvement activities—especially as they apply to the leadership process itself.

Human resources management. An organization must have an adequate number of competent clinical and support staff (including volunteers, if applicable) available to carry out all key governance, management, clinical, and support processes to fulfill its objectives, including continuous improvement efforts. As in all personnel management areas, staff performance must be regularly assessed and improved through continuing education and training opportunities. Continuous feedback on the performance of critical functions is essential for quality improvement.

Information management. High-quality ambulatory care depends on timely, valid, and reliable information about

- the patient being served, his or her care, and treatment results;
- management and business functions;
- the performance of the organization as a whole;
- other organizations' performance from external reference databases, if available; and
- knowledge of emerging clinical pathways and best practices.

It is essential that an organization meet these information needs to coordinate, integrate, assess, and improve services.

Improving organization performance. Organizations that excel evaluate themselves rigorously and continually strive to improve. These organizations are balanced between the demands of everyday functions (for example, handling daily patient load) and the need for continuous organization improvement. With planning, organizations can create well-designed processes, measure the performance of existing processes, assess processes based on the measurement data, and improve outcomes by redesigning existing processes or by designing new processes when necessary. The Joint Commission's improving organization performance standards are compatible with a variety of process improvement methodologies. Many of these methodologies share the following key concepts:

- *Assessment of customer satisfaction and experience.* It is essential to consider the patients' judgments about quality, their views on the need for improvement, and their experiences with care.
- *Technology and environment of care measurement.* Processes must be in place to evaluate the facilities, equipment, machinery, and supplies used in care delivery.
- *Research and knowledge building.* Searching should be continuous for better and more efficient ways to perform functions and processes.
- *Systematic performance improvement.* Close coordination and collaboration are necessary among organization units (for example, clinical, customer service, billing, data entry, or clerical staff), services, and disciplines.
- *Process focus.* Improvement opportunities are usually found in processes, not in an individual clinician's performance.

Cycle for Improving Performance

An organization must have a systematic approach to improvement. The cycle for improving performance—the third component of this framework—describes such an approach. This cycle is anchored in the real work of an organization—the functions and processes it carries out every day to pursue its goals and mission. This cycle can be carried out by existing work groups as part of everyday activities.

When the processes or functions being addressed cross service, discipline, or departmental boundaries, it is especially helpful to form a representative team composed of the people who have ownership of the process, who are responsible for the process, who carry out the process, and who are affected by the process. Cross-functional and cross-discipline processes are considered especially important because they are often the basis of improving organization performance in ambulatory care organizations.

To improve processes and outcomes over time, staff of ambulatory care organizations (working from a known set of objectives and mission) must systemati-

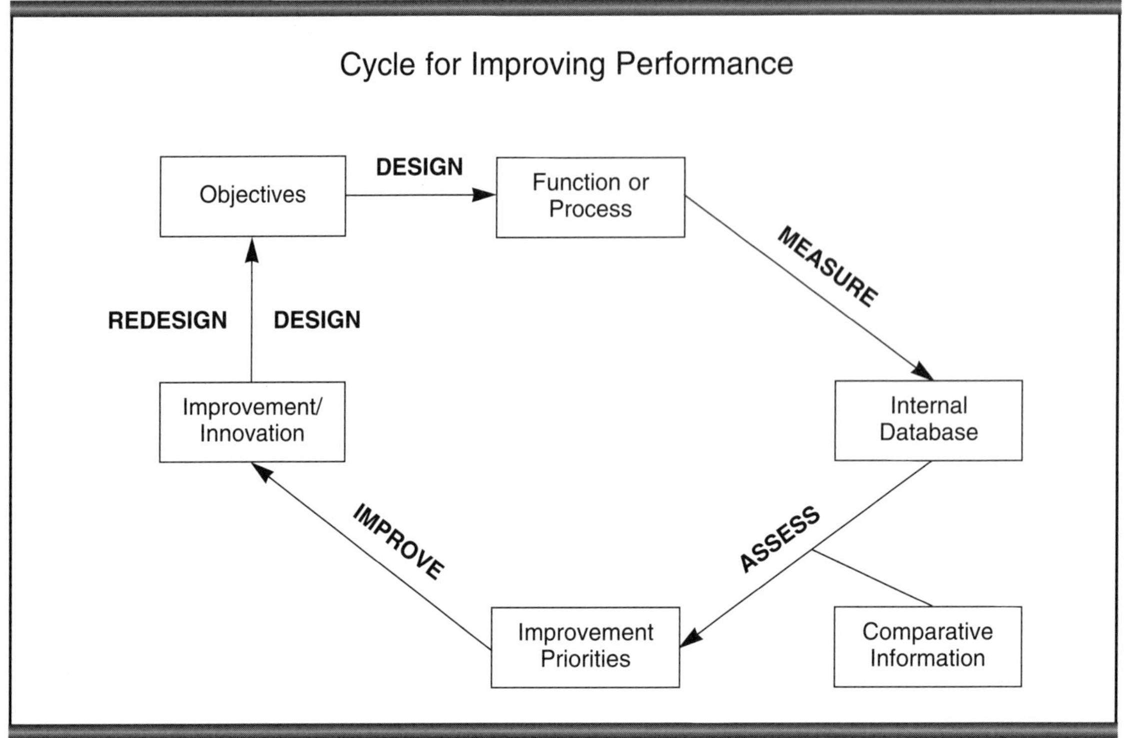

Figure 1-2. This cycle is composed of activities (represented by the arrows) and their related inputs and outputs (in boxes).

cally and scientifically design, measure, assess, and improve these processes and outcomes.

Figure 1-2, above, describes the building blocks of the improvement cycle. As its cyclical nature suggests, performance improvement is a continuous process. Specific tenets of the cycle include the following:

- *Objectives* for achieving a clear goal or purpose are necessary before launching a design effort;
- A design effort results in a *function or process*—that is, a related series of activities directed toward accomplishing a specific goal;
- Measuring performance of a function or process results in an *internal database,* which is used to establish baseline data and to assess performance over time;
- One of the tools used to assess performance is *comparative information* from other sources, such as reference databases, practice guidelines, and best practices;

- Assessment of a process should result in identifying *opportunities for improvement* and setting priorities; and
- Based on these priorities, the organization creates, tests, and implements specific *improvements and innovations,* which involve redesign or a new design, respectively, of a process or function.

The cycle continues even after it has been completed for a given function or process for the first time. The objectives are viewed, reviewed, and perhaps changed again; new information is gathered from a similar facility using a similar process. Simultaneously, measurement continues to determine whether improvement has occurred and can be sustained, and the internal database continues to grow. Assessment and evaluation using cumulative information may identify further opportunities for improvement.

The improvement cycle is truly a model for understanding organization change. Hence, it may be applied at any level of generality or specificity. For example, *function* could refer to the entire ambulatory care organization or it could refer to a multidisciplinary, cross-service activity (such as patient assessment or treatment planning). *Process* could refer to a number of clinical activities (for example, how family members are instructed to care for their asthmatic child or how physicians prescribe drugs for hypertensive patients). Process may also refer to support and managerial tasks (for example, how new staff receive appropriate orientation).

Subsequent chapters of this book provide more in-depth explanation of these concepts and improvement appraisals, and specific examples of how to carry out this cycle.

Relationship of the Cycle to the Joint Commission's Standards

The cycle for improving organization performance is the basis of the Joint Commission's improving organization performance standards. Please refer to these standards, their intent statements and their scoring guidelines in your most current copy of the *Comprehensive Accreditation Manual for Ambulatory Care.* The standards, like the cycle, focus primarily on the performance of an organization's systems and processes, not solely on performance of individuals.

Reference

1996 Comprehensive Accreditation Manual for Ambulatory Care. Oakbrook Terrace, IL: Joint Commission, 1996.

CHAPTER 2: Design

Chapter Highlights

Why Do We Design?

Design requires setting objectives based on

- the organization's mission, vision, and plans;
- the needs and expectations of the individuals served, staff, and others;
- current knowledge about organization and clinical activities;
- relevant data about performance and outcomes; and
- availability of resources.

What Do We Design?

- Design focuses on functions and processes.

How Do We Design?

- Successful designs are created by using a systematic method, basing decisions on data, involving the right people, and finding the best information.

Who Creates the Design?

- Leaders set priorities for design.
- The process's owners, suppliers, and customers create the design with other expert individuals as necessary.

Examples of Design

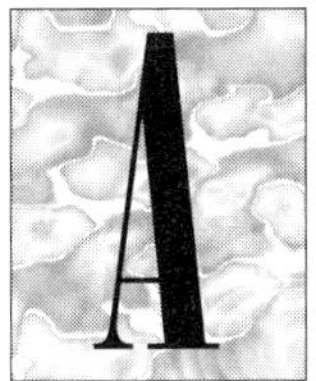

ssessing and diagnosing a patient, referring a patient to a specialist, designing wellness education, creating and implementing a care plan for a child with asthma, implementing a computerized information system, establishing an infrastructure for performance improvement—no single activity, process, or function in an ambulatory care organization is an end in itself, but each is a necessary component of a larger whole. Each activity is designed to fulfill a specific objective and is carefully interwoven into the organization structure.

When reviewing the organization, office, branch, department, program, service, team, or individual level of performance, each ambulatory care professional needs to regularly stop and ask two vital questions:

- What goals are we trying to accomplish?
- How can we best accomplish these goals?

These questions are the essence of the design concept. The design component of the cycle for improving performance focuses on determining specific objectives of organization activities and developing, designing, and implementing functions and processes to achieve those objectives.

As ambulatory care organizations attempt to improve customer service and stay competitive, many are designing and offering new services or redesigning their present services to be more efficient and "customer friendly" and to produce better care outcomes. Some of the current processes and functions in ambulatory care organizations reflect local policy, response to regulatory pressure, or administrative directives, rather than following a carefully integrated design.

Figure 2-1, page 28, illustrates how design fits into the cycle for improving performance. The inputs for design are organization objectives; leaders must decide what they want the new design to accomplish. Design activities can involve multiple phases, each of which may include some measurement and benchmarking to ensure that the project is proceeding as planned; if appropriate modifications should be made.

Many of the same techniques apply to designing a new process and redesigning an existing process (for example, reviewing state-of-the-art knowledge about the process). However, it is important to distinguish between *design* and *redesign*. Design creates new processes—in effect, starting with a clean slate. *Redesign* takes a fresh look at an existing process—in effect, revising and improving the process. For example, to redesign a process, an organization would use

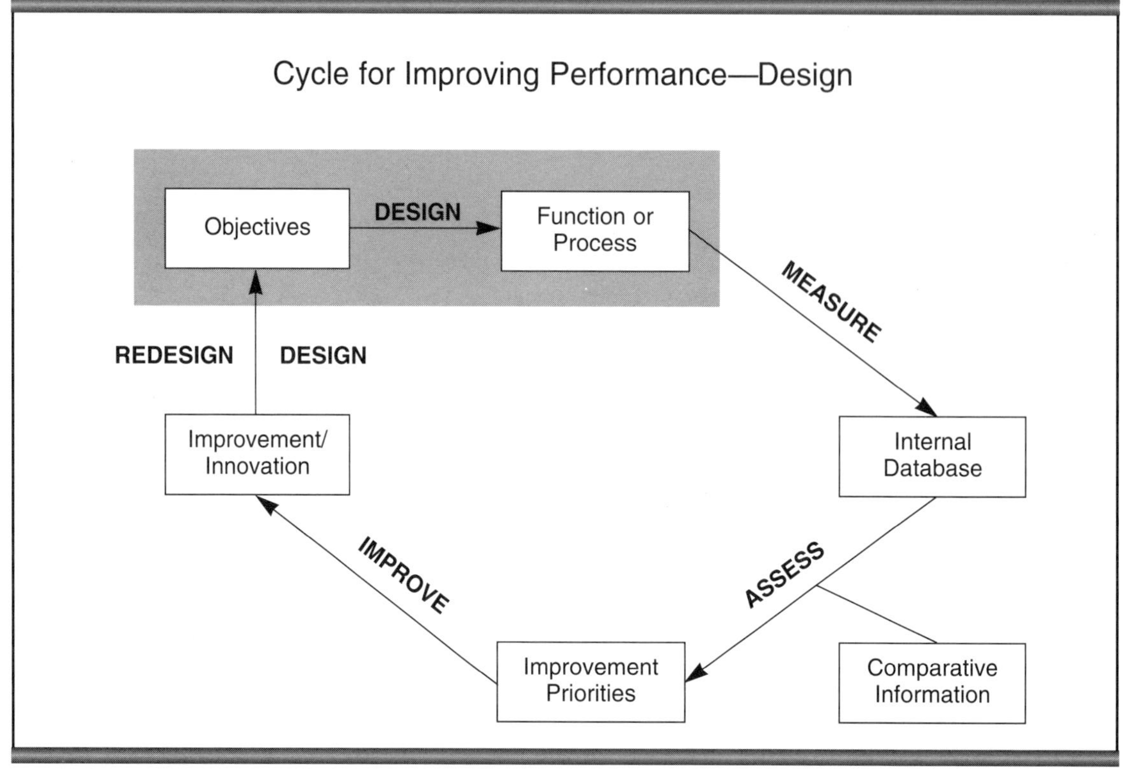

Figure 2-1. This figure highlights the design stage of the improvement cycle.

information about its current performance of the process. In contrast, organization creating a new design would not have that information to use, because the process would not yet exist. Both processes can be very helpful in driving improvement efforts.

This chapter focuses primarily on the design of new activities; for example, opening a clinic in a new community, extending a product line (such as endoscopy), or offering new clinical services (such as diabetes management).

Why Do We Design? Setting Objectives

Organization objectives and processes are intrinsically tied together through design. To be successful, an ambulatory care organization must set goals related to its mission, vision, and values. Organization processes should reflect these goals. Unfortunately, in many contemporary health care organizations, the objectives of a process are often unwritten and unspoken, resulting in less effective work processes. As we approach the concept of design, all activities should be regularly examined for their relevance, value, feasibility, and effectiveness.

Such an examination may be accomplished using existing everyday work tasks (for example, assessing a patient who arrives at a clinic with flu symptoms). This examination may cause the organization's leaders to conclude that a new process is needed or that an existing process needs to be redesigned. Therefore, organizations should have a systematic process in place for

- reviewing organization goals and the activities that fulfill them;
- reviewing and selecting opportunities that require a new design effort;
- designing new processes or functions; and
- measuring and assessing the new process or function.

This systematic process helps an organization identify opportunities for innovation. It also provides a method to fairly weigh the benefits and drawbacks of a newly designed process or function. In addition, it provides a method to involve the right people at the start and get the best knowledge for creating the design. Finally, it helps leaders determine whether the results of the design effort meet the objectives.

Organization goals are not created in isolation. Development of an organization's goals and the design of activities to pursue those goals requires an organization leaders to ask:

- Is this process, function, or service consistent with the organization's mission, vision, and other plans?
- What do the organization's patients, staff, and other customers expect from the process, function, or service?
- How do they think it should work?
- What do scientific and professional experts and other reliable sources say about the design process or function?
- What information is available about the performance of similar processes, functions, or services in other organizations?

The answers to these questions help the organization develop a basic set of performance expectations that guide process design as well as measurement and assessment of the process, function, or service.

Mission, Vision, and Plans

Any design should consider how the resulting process or function will serve the organization's

- mission,
- future vision, and
- plans for carrying out its mission and fulfilling its vision.

The mission, vision, and plans of the organization answer the basic question "What is the organization for?" One of the best methods to define an organization's work is in relation to its primary activities. An environmental assessment is also an important source of information when establishing mission, vision, and plans, and when analyzing whether current activities are fulfilling an organization's overall strategic plan. Such data help leaders determine how the vision of the organization (in the future) will serve the community. For example, a community health center might learn that the management of pediatric asthma is a priority. Or a primary care clinic might learn that it needs to recruit more nurses. These elements (that is, mission, vision, plans) are also important for the organization to develop a shared sense of identity and culture.

Needs, Expectations, and Experiences of Individuals Served, Staff, and Others

To design successful processes and functions yielding better outcomes, ambulatory care organizations must understand the needs, expectations, and experiences of patients and their families.

A comprehensive community-based needs assessment has been a tenet of ambulatory care practice for years. The patients and their families are the primary consumers of the ambulatory health care services. Meeting their needs is critical to the organization's survival. Once these needs, expectations, and experiences are understood, the organization can decide how and to what extent they can be met.

Equally important are the internal customers—the organization's clinical and support staff and volunteers who will carry out processes. Organization goals must also reflect their needs and expectations. Understanding the perspective of internal customers within an organization can be quite useful and can help all staff work in a collaborative manner and become more attuned to each other's needs and expectations. Other important customers and suppliers to consider in this process are purchasers, payers, physicians, referral sources, accreditors, regulators, and the community as a whole.

Discussing the nine dimensions of performance (see page 12) with specific groups is an excellent way to elicit needs and expectations. This can be accomplished using focus groups or sampling from existing committees or advisory groups. As these data become available, measures can be established to determine whether the services provided fulfill those needs and expectations.

Current Knowledge About Organization and Clinical Activities

Improvement requires knowledge. An organization's goals—and any activities designed to pursue those goals—must consider the best knowledge available concerning management and clinical activities. If, for example, a community health center is considering increasing the frequency with which preventive tests, such as Pap smears, are performed or if it is thinking about offering alternative or holistic services to patients (for example, chiropractic), it should consider both current practices within the organization and other existing state-of-the-art practices. Such knowledge is available from expert sources both inside and outside an organization, including other ambulatory care organizations, other health care organizations with similar processes, professional literature, professional societies, trade associations, and consultants.

Likewise, expert knowledge of current practices is crucial in the design of any clinical- or individual-focused care activities. Contemporary clinical knowledge can be found in information on clinical pathways, parameters of care, scientific and research literature, practice guidelines, and standards of care. Several examples throughout this book show ambulatory care organizations using subject matter expertise as a tool for successful design and improvement.

Relevant Data

Data are the cornerstone of successful design and improvement efforts. The importance of valid, reliable data and its effective use, cannot be overemphasized. For example, a primary care clinic would not decide to introduce a new scheduling system without first gathering data about patient volume at various times that the clinic is open.

For redesign and other improvement efforts, information about care outcomes is especially valuable. Outcomes data should encompass both specific performance within the organization (for example, aggregate data showing historical rates of specific outcomes for specific diagnoses) and information from existing reference databases. Information from reference databases (compiled by professional or trade associations, ambulatory care systems, payers, regulatory agencies, the Joint Commission, and others) can help ambulatory care organizations determine their goals for individual patients and patient populations. Existing health services research information is an added resource in this area. Use of aggregate and summary data in performance improvement efforts is described in more detail in Chapter 3.

Availability of Resources

In the current climate, ambulatory care organizations are painfully aware that their resources (that is, money, space, time, and staff) are limited. Limited financial resources have affected many areas, including staffing levels and salaries, equipment purchases, and length of time physicians can spend with patients. Funding cuts have also spawned innovative treatment approaches such as telemedicine and on-line patient education.

Nonetheless, every organization seeks ways to control costs and improve efficiency without sacrificing quality or essential services. In their short- and long-range planning, organizations face daunting decisions as they compare their mission and vision with their available resources. Organizations contemplating new design efforts must weigh the availability of resources against the potential benefits to the patient and for the organization. Ideally, quality planning and business planning can be integrated to provide cost/benefit analysis for critical decisions. The visionary leader's dreams and the operations manager's pragmatic warnings need to be reconciled with current resources.

What Do We Design? Functions and Processes

When addressing what to design, think in terms of the everyday work of the organization. This work can be defined in terms of numerous functions and processes. Stated another way, what is actually created, provided, or conducted by the organization?

As described in Chapter 1, a *function* is a group of processes with a common goal. A *process* is a series of linked, goal-directed activities. For example, function could refer to a multidisciplinary, cross-service activity, such as, assessment, care treatment, medication monitoring, and education. A process can be a clinical activity, such as the systematic way a physician assesses a patient's medical history, symptoms, and life-style. A process can also refer to an administrative or operational activity, such as the specific steps taken to verify a patient's insurance or refer a patient to a specialist.

How Do We Design?

Any new process design must pay careful attention to the customer-supplier relationships inherent in the process. The design should facilitate the greatest efficiency in these relationships, coordinating and integrating all relevant activities to produce desirable outcomes.

To create a new design for care delivery, management, or support processes, organizations should consider the following process design guidelines:

- ***Design a systematic method to determine the effect of the process on the organization's mission, vision, plans, customers, resources, and so forth.*** Questionnaires, informal discussions, focus groups, and consensus techniques are useful tools.
- ***Base decisions on valid, reliable data.*** Data are the key to developing accurate design specifications and to assessing the effectiveness of the design.
- ***Involve the right people.*** Any design effort should include representatives of all groups who are responsible for and participate in the process, including the individuals served (that is, all process owners).
- ***Strategically review a variety of information on the subject.*** Examine the professional literature, advice of professional societies or trade associations, and practices of other organizations. A view of other organizations' practices and experiences can also help prevent mistakes and inspire creative thinking.

Several additional building blocks relevant to the design process include the following:

- Understanding patient needs, expectations, and preferences;
- Reviewing the type and nature of care delivered; and
- Being knowledgeable of the organization design, structure, and work processes.

Who Creates the Design?

All staff participate in the design process. The Joint Commission's leadership standards require that leaders and managers take an active role in overseeing and setting priorities for design. Generally, managers are responsible for processes within their areas; design of processes with a wider scope may be overseen by managers. In small facilities, the entire staff might be intricately involved in the design process.

Design and redesign efforts require resources, including money, time, and appropriate equipment and support. Leaders must ensure that the staff involved have the necessary resources and expertise to accomplish their task. Further, their authority to make changes should be commensurate with their responsibility for process improvements. Although regular feedback and contact with management are important, rigid control can stifle creativity. A good balance of guidance and direction with ample freedom and systematic feedback is indicated.

The group that creates the process should include the people responsible for the process, the staff who will carry out the process, and the staff affected by the process. If appropriate, the group members could include staff from different services, different disciplines, and different job categories. When the group needs a perspective not offered by its representatives, it should conduct interviews or surveys outside the group or invite new members into the work group.

Examples of Design

Example 2-1: Developing a Patient Education Program at a University-Based Student Health Services

The Setting and Background

Ruffin University is a hypothetical university in an Indiana city with approximately 10,000 students. The student health services is owned and managed by the university. It provides primary care services to the student population. When emergencies arise or speciality care is needed, students are sent to the local hospital five miles from the university. An administrator, a primary care physician, two registered nurses, and two secretaries are employed full-time at the clinic. In addition, medical residents from the local hospital help out at the clinic each day. Student workers are also employed on a part-time basis to help with administrative tasks.

In January 1997, Tina O'Malley, the clinic administrator, learns that her budget for the coming school year (1997-1998) will be cut by 7½% due to cuts in state funds for education. In the past, Ruffin has maintained a student population at approximately 10,000 students. Due to the state and federal funding cutbacks, university administration felt it necessary to accept 500 new students for the upcoming fall semesters to increase revenues.

Tina and other university department directors are asked to develop plans to manage the budget reductions and increased student population by May. The plans will then be approved by the administration and implemented over the summer break in time for the fall quarter.

Example Highlights

Setting:
Ruffin University Student Health Services, Anycity, Indiana

Performance Improvement Initiative:
Patient education program to reduce unnecessary access to student health services.

Dimensions of Performance Addressed:
Availability, efficiency, timeliness.

Comments:
This example illustrates how a team using total quality management/continuous quality improvement (TQM/CQI) tools and principles develops a patient education program. The Joint Commission framework for performance improvement is compatible with many improvement methodologies, including TQM/CQI.

The Problem

Worried about how the present clinic staff is going to provide care to more students on a reduced budget, Tina calls a staff meeting one morning. She explains that the number of students that access the clinic during the 1997-1998 year will increase by 5% (15 more students a week on average), and asks for ideas on how to accommodate the increase.

A few seconds of silence pass before the clinic staff starts brainstorming ideas, such as getting more residents to help out and extending clinic hours.

"Those ideas might help us meet the increased number of students," Tina says. "However, because of our budget cuts, we do not have the extra staff to manage the additional residents, or run the clinic during off hours. The only way I see to meet this challenge is to decrease the number of students who access the health services."

"You mean by keeping students healthy?" asks Todd Cunningham, MD, the physician director.

"Ideally, yes. Plus, we can try to cut the number of students who come to us unnecessarily for minor ailments. You guys are always complaining that you spend most of your time treating students for runny noses. Let's cut the number of students who come to us unnecessarily by teaching them how to manage those minor ailments at home."

"We barely have time to treat students who come to us," says Todd. "How are we going to find time to sponsor a major patient education campaign?"

Tina agrees that time is scarce and appoints a project team to determine the appropriate solution. All staff will be expected to help the team as needed. "Right now, we only need to design a patient education solution that cuts the percentage of patients who access the system by 5%," she says. "However, this solution should not be a one-time thing. Hopefully, it can be developed so we can continue to educate students on various health topics."

After some discussion, the clinic staff formulate a problem statement: "Develop a method for increasing student awareness of simple self-care management so as to reduce the percentage of students who unnecessarily access the health services by 5% in 1997 and 1998. This tool should be expandable into a long-term patient education resource for students."

The Project Team

Three clinic staff are assigned to serve on the project team: the physician director, a registered nurse, and a secretary. A resident and a student employee also volunteer to serve on the team. Tina is the team's leader and oversees each meeting. In addition, the university assigns a graduate student from the business school to help facilitate the meetings. The team meets on a weekly basis for eight weeks with several half-day retreats to allow for a more intensive working phase.

Before the first meeting, Tina meets with the graduate student facilitator, Fred Savon. Fred is well versed in TQM/CQI principles and thinks the team might benefit from following such an approach. Tina has a general understanding of the TQM/CQI concepts from her business training and agrees that these concepts might help achieve better results. However, she explains that they do not have time to train the team in these principles.

Fred suggests using TQM/CQI concepts and tools on a "just-in-time" basis. At the first meeting, Fred could give a half-hour explanation of the basic principles of TQM, such as customer thinking. Then, whenever the team got stuck or might benefit from TQM know-how, Fred could suggest a concept or tool that might help. For example, he might teach them how to create a flowchart when outlining the steps in a newly designed process.

See page 104 for a discussion on flowcharts.

Tina likes Fred's idea, but she asks that he not use the terms "TQM" or "CQI." "Just call them 'some basic management principles,'" she suggests. "The team has enough to accomplish. I don't want them worried about learning a whole new management approach as well."

The Design Process

Defining the problem. After Fred gives an overview of TQM/CQI at the first team meeting, Tina suggests that the team begin by further defining the problem. She asks the group to brainstorm on ways that students unnecessarily access the student health system.

This discussion yields a list of items, including:

- Many students come to us for minor colds and headaches—things they can treat themselves.
- We see a lot of the same patients all the time.
- A lot of students come for birth control.
- Some students wait until they get really sick to come to us.
- A lot of health problems we treat result from students who don't eat right or take care of themselves.
- Students exacerbate flu or cold symptoms by going out drinking or staying up all night studying.
- Many student complaints are related to behavioral health problems, like anxiety over tests, homesickness, depression, and so forth.
- We treat a lot of sexually transmitted diseases that could have been prevented.

- Many students don't know what the student health services does or how we operate.
- They come to us for things they should go to the hospital emergency room for and vice versa.

At this point, Fred describes the Pareto principle to the team. "Eighty percent of trouble comes from 20% of the problems," he says. "If you can determine the 'vital few' reasons that students misuse the health care system, then you can begin to get at the heart of the problem."

See page 107 for a discussion on Pareto charts.

The team discusses how to determine the major reasons students misuse the system. They decide to look at patient records from the previous school year. Alice Moyer, a registered nurse, and Phil Jector, a student employee, volunteer for the task. To get a good cross-sample, the team suggests reviewing records for one-week periods in October, January, and April.

Narrowing the cause. At the next meeting, Alice and Phil present their findings. Of the 143 students seen in the three weeks of the study:

- 57 students had come for causes that required physician care. These varied from severe flu symptoms to annual checkups.
- 34 students had come for minor cold symptoms. As expected, a large percentage of these patients were seen in January as opposed to October and April.
- 22 students had come in for other symptoms that could be treated at home, such as minor back pain or hay fever.
- 18 students had wanted to talk about birth control options.
- 12 students had come for various other reasons.

When placed in a Pareto chart (see Figure 2-2, page 39), the team could easily see that they should concentrate on educating students about how to treat cold symptoms on their own. However, they concluded that a larger patient education effort aimed at helping students identify and treat various ailments at home would be even more beneficial.

Student focus groups. At this point, Todd suggests that they develop and distribute a small booklet outlining at-home treatments for colds and other common, nonserious ailments to all students. "That's a good idea," says Tina. "But we

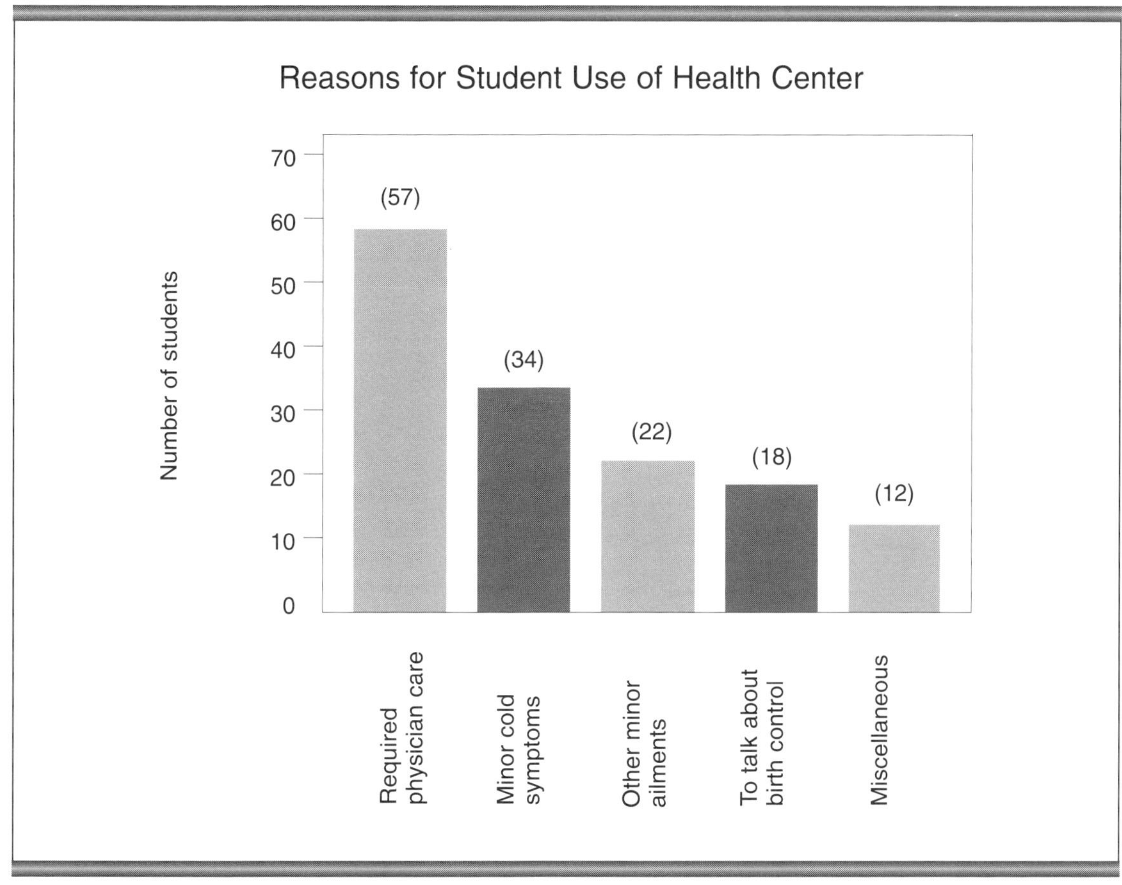

Figure 2-2. Of the 143 students seen at Ruffin Student Health Services, 56 sought care for minor cold symptoms and other minor ailments that they could treat themselves at home.

need to find out what type of intervention would work the best. The only way to do that is to ask the students."

At Fred's suggestion, the team decides to conduct focus groups with students to find out the best way to disseminate self-care information. The focus groups includes students who had recently accessed the health service for minor ailments, as well as students chosen at random from various graduating classes, sexes, and races.

Focus group participants are told that the student health services hopes to develop a patient education tool that helps students assume treatment of minor ailments on their own. Participants are asked what they want and need in such a patient education tool. Student suggestions include:

- I need to be able to find information easily. I don't want to have to learn medical terms. I want to be able to look up 'fever' and find out what to do.
- I need specific instructions, like do A, B, and C.
- I want to be sure that all the instructions have been approved by physicians and are up to date.
- The language should be easy to understand.
- It should be explicit about when I should see a doctor. Like, if a cold lasts over a week, should I go to the clinic?
- What if I have a question after reading the self-care instructions? I still want to be able to talk to a doctor if I need to.

Using the students' feedback, the team identifies the following six features that they want to include in the patient education tool:

- Information should be organized by symptoms.
- Specific, step-by-step instructions should be given in layperson's terms.
- Material should be physician approved.
- Information should be easy to update and distribute.
- Tool should allow for interactivity between clinicians and students.
- Method should be inexpensive.

Benchmarking. Tina asks Todd and Mary O'Toole, a resident, to benchmark other self-care programs at various types of health care organizations across the country.

See page 96 for a discussion on benchmarking.

They research current literature and identify three types of self-care programs, including:

- Self-care books distributed to patients;
- Telephone triage systems where patients call a hotline staffed by nurses who provide self-care instructions based on the patient's symtoms;
- On-line programs via a hospital's or university's home page on the Internet's World Wide Web. These programs include patient education, discussion groups on health topics, and other resources.

Patient Education Tools Evaluated Against Criteria

Criteria	Self-care Book	Telephone Triage System	On-line Resource
Organized by symptoms	✔	✔	✔
Provides specific, step-by-step instructions in layperson's terms	✔	✔	✔
Material is physician approved	✔	✔	✔
Easy to update and distribute		✔	✔
Allows for interaction between clinicians and students		✔	✔
Inexpensive			✔

Figure 2-3. To determine which patient education resource best met their objectives, student health services staff compared various tools against six predetermined criteria.

Todd and Mary interview several organizations that are using various tools and present the pros and cons of each tool at a team meeting. Based on their research, the team completes a matrix comparing each tool against the six features, or criteria, they identified (see Figure 2-3, above).

See page 108 for a discussion on selection grids.

From this comparison, the team identifies the on-line patient education resource as meeting all their criteria. The telephone triage system comes close, but it would be too expensive to staff. A self-care book would be too expensive and difficult to update, and it would not allow for interaction between clinicians and students.

The team agrees that an on-line resource would allow them to easily distribute to patients materials that gave specific, step-by-step instructions. Also, they could include discussion groups and e-mail features that allow students and clinicians to interact. Finally, the overhead costs for developing such a resource would be low. Few materials would need to be printed and distributed. The university had already developed a home page on the Internet's World Wide Web.

Graduate computer science students were offering assistance on how to add information to the home page.

Determining computerization ability. The team agrees that the on-line self-help program would probably meet their objectives. However, they are concerned that only students with access to a computer and a modem would be able to use the system.

Tina points out that Ruffin University is farther ahead than other universities in terms of computerization. All students are advised to bring a computer to school. Also, students who do not have a computer can use one of the 500 computers the university has set up in dorms, the library, and the student union.

Phil, the student employee, agrees. "I don't know anyone who doesn't use a computer at least every few days. Most people answer as many e-mails as phone calls."

Despite Tina's and Phil's confidence, the other team members are hesitant to begin developing an on-line resource before they can be sure students will use it. To help answer their concerns, they develop a short survey:

- Do you own a computer with a modem?
- If you do not own a computer and modem, do you have easy access to such equipment?
- If you came down with a cold and knew you could find instructions on-line on how to treat it, would you access that information before coming to the student health services?
- If you had the choice between accessing health information on-line or from a book or a pamphlet, which would you prefer? Why?

The team distributes the survey to all freshmen and sophomores enrolled in required English classes. Students are asked to fill out the survey in class; 47% respond to the survey.

The results reveal that

- of respondents, 42% own a computer and a modem, and another 36% have easy access to such technology. Ten percent do not have easy access to a computer, and 12% did not answer the question (see Figure 2-4, page 43).

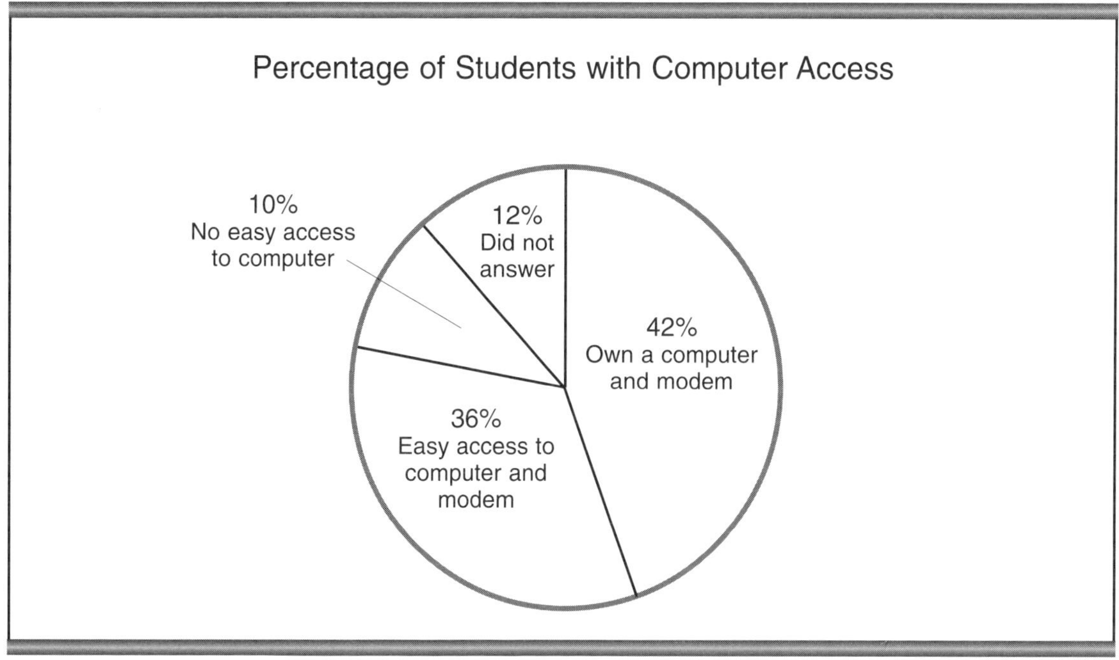

Figure 2-4. Before implementing an on-line patient education resource for students, the student health services surveyed students to see if they owned or had access to a computer. The majority of students (78%) reported either owning or having easy access to such technology.

- a large majority of respondents (72%) say they would access an on-line resource for health information. Thirteen percent say they would not, 8% say they did not know, and 7% did not answer the question.
- seventy percent of the students prefer an on-line resource and 30% prefer a book or pamphlet. Those who prefer the on-line resource gave many reasons why, including "I have to cart around enough books," and "The on-line resource would allow me to ask questions via e-mail." Students who prefer a book or pamphlet said so primarily because they like having printed materials to refer to.

Based on the results of the survey, the team decides to implement the on-line patient education resource. However, team members realize that they need to stage a marketing campaign that will inform students about the service as well as convince them to use it. They also want to make sure students know they can print or download any on-line material so they have written materials to refer to.

Putting the Plan into Action

After receiving administration approval, the team spends the summer quarter developing the materials to put on the health center's on-line service. Two graduate students help full-time with the project as part of their thesis work—a computer science student handles the technology and a public relations student helps write patient education materials in a user-friendly manner. The final product includes:

- Four symptom-based algorithms that give students step-by-step directions on how to treat the following complaints: fever, cough, common cold symptoms, and sore throat.
- A list of tips on how to prevent colds and flu.
- Links to other Internet World Wide Web sites that contain helpful health information.
- "Ask the Doctor," includes answers to 20 common health questions, including how to protect against sexually transmitted diseases. Students can add additional questions and the physician director will answer each question within three working days.
- E-mail to the clinic. Twice a day, the registered nurse and the physician director will take time to respond to students' specific questions.

To determine whether the resource is successful, the team identifies four performance measures that it will track over the first year of implementation:

See page 69 for a discussion on indicators.

- Number of students who use the on-line resource per month.
- Number of students who access the student health services per month.
- Percentage of students who access the student health services for common cold, flu, cough, and sore throat symptoms.
- Student satisfaction with the on-line resource (as measured by a semi-annual survey).

Depending on the success of the on-line resource, clinic staff hope to expand the site with additional health information. They plan to add many more algorithms that advise students on how to treat ailments such as low back pain and skin rashes. They also hope to sponsor a weekly on-line discussion group that focuses on "hot" health topics.

Example 2-2. Developing a Credentialing Process at a Health Maintenance Organization

The Setting and Background

In the past, licensed independent practitioners (LIPs) who applied to be a member of Quincy Care Network's provider panel had been asked for limited information concerning their credentials (such as licensure and malpractice insurer). Leaders of this hypothetical, mid-sized health maintenance organization (HMO) in Idaho had always relied on hospitals to handle credentialing of its providers. Physicians and other LIPs who applied to Quincy Care Network were asked whether they were affiliated with a hospital. If they were, the HMO assumed that the hospital had already credentialed the LIP and that, therefore, he or she was competent.

However, early in 1996, leaders began to realize that this approach was no longer sufficient. To obtain employer contracts, they wanted to ensure the competency of their physician members.

Leaders of Quincy Care Network recruited Sally Hopkins from a local hospital to serve as Quincy Care Network's new Credentialing Supervisor. She is expected to set up a credentialing process within eight months. Sarah Riley, the adminis-trative assistant who has handled the processing of physician applications for the last two years, will serve as Sally's assistant.

Example Highlights

Setting:
Quincy Care Network, Any town, Idaho

Performance Improvement Initiative:
Develop a cost-effective credentialing system that ensures competent LIPs and incorporates performance improvement information in the reappointment process.

Dimensions of Performance Addressed:
Continuity, effectivenss, efficacy.

Comments:
This example illustrates how staff first identified the intended outcome of a system, and then determined what needed to be accomplished.

Designing the Process

Defining the goals of the process. Sally spends her first few weeks on the job trying to learn what Quincy wants to achieve from the credentialing process. She and Sarah study Quincy Care Network's mission, vision, and strategic plan. In addition, they meet with various HMO leaders and staff and ask them what they expect from the credentialing process. From these conversations, Sally concludes that leaders want to:

- Develop a defined process for appointing, reappointing, and privileging LIPs to ensure their competence;
- Develop mechanisms to incorporate performance improvement information (for example, utilization information, patient outcomes, compliance with clinical guidelines) into the reappointment of physicians;
- Use the credentialing and privileging process as an opportunity to gather additional data about LIPs (for example, office addresses, hours of operation);
- Create a database on all LIPs that can be used for appointment and verification, as well as other functions, such as contracting, marketing, health research, and so forth; and
- Work toward a paperless system that uses automation to simplify and increase cost- efficiency of credentialing and privileging.

Sally and Sarah present this list of objectives to Quincy leaders who enthusiastically agree with the objectives and request they draw up an estimate of the required resources to implement the credentialing process.

Recruiting internal expertise. Sally states that one of the first resources she needs to draw on is the internal expertise of staff, including staff from quality improvement, risk management and utilization review, marketing, and information management. Leaders identify individuals who can provide such knowledge and assign them to a team under Sally's direction. In addition, leaders ask Phyllis Sedgewick, the quality improvement director, to serve as facilitator.

Identifying the macro process. At their first meeting, the team members discuss the draft objectives. Phyllis suggests that team members begin by defining the major steps in a credentialing system. Sally describes how credentialing is typi-

See page 104 for a discussion on flowcharts.

cally carried out while Phyllis draws a macro flowchart on a flip chart that encompasses the major steps Sally identifies.

Once these steps are identified, other team members suggest ways the process could be simplified or expanded to meet the team's objectives. The marketing manager suggests that LIPs supply additional information on their credentialing application, such as their office hours. The information systems manager identifies areas of the process that could be easily automated.

By the end of the meeting, the task force has developed a macro flowchart for the appointment process (see Figure 2-5, page 48). The committee spends the next few meetings developing additional flowcharts for granting of privileges and for reappointment.

Determining what to do first. The task force members then review the flowcharts they have created. At Phyllis' suggestion, the team develops a Gantt chart (see Figure 2-6, page 49) that spells outs the tasks that need to be accomplished.

They begin by brainstorming the various tasks that need to be completed to implement each step in the process.

Then, the team determines what tasks need to be completed. By the end of the meeting, they have a detailed summary of what tasks need to be accomplished by what date and by whom.

The team then identifies two tasks that must be accomplished in the next few weeks:

- Developing a draft credentialing application, which includes identifying the information that needs to be obtained from LIPs when they apply for initial appointment; and
- Identifying a commercial software program that Quincy can use to develop a database of all LIPs and to ease the burden of the verification process.

Sally and Sarah are assigned responsibility for developing the application. Doug Baron, the IS director, is asked to investigate various software programs that will meet Quincy's needs.

Developing the application. Sally and Sarah begin by brainstorming a list of information that is typically asked of LIPs during credentialing. They compare this list with Joint Commission's standards and state and federal regulations to

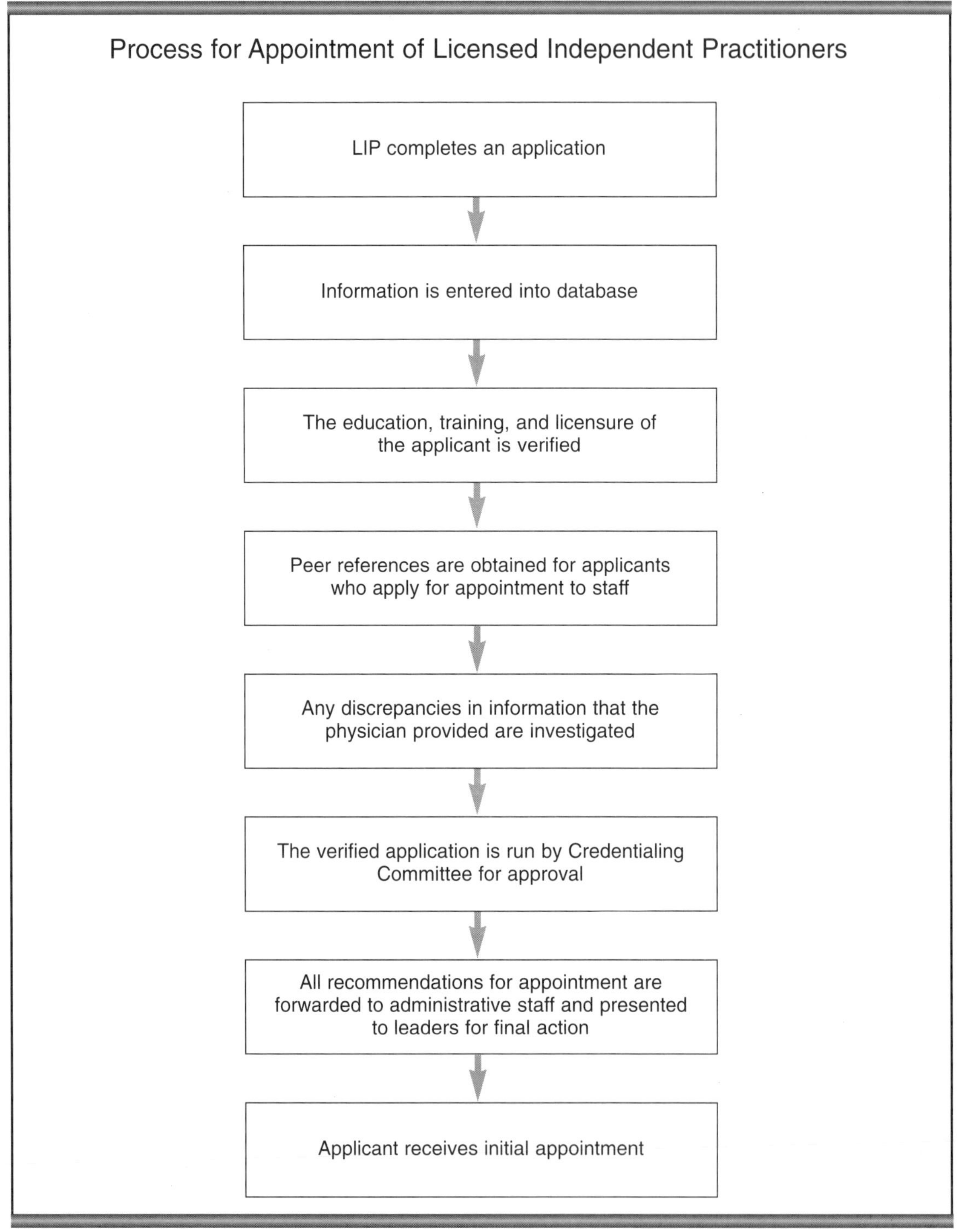

Figure 2-5. Quincy's credentialing design team began by developing a flowchart of the typical steps in the appointment process.

Competency and Privileging Process

Task	Person(s) Responsible	Apr	May	Jun	Jul	Aug	Sep	Oct	Nov	Dec	Jan–June
DESIGN PHASE											
Develop credentialing application	SH and SR										
Develop appropriate software package	RB										
Define policies and procedures that outline appointment, reappointment, and privileging process	SH and SR										
Identify and appoint credentialing committee	SH										
Develop informational materials for all Quincy staff and providers describing new process	LA										
Determine staffing needs in credentialing office	SH										
Set up and test necessary information systems	RB and SR										
Develop press releases informing employer groups and other contractors of credentialing	PZ										
Identify performance measures	SH and SR										
IMPLEMENTATION PHASE											
Pilot	Team										
Assess process agains performance measures	Team										
Make necessary improvements	Team										

Figure 2-6. To help determine what tasks to undertake in what order, the credentialing design team developed a Gantt chart that detailed who needed to accomplish which task by a certain date.

ensure it meets all external requirements. The result is a lengthy list of information that must be requested from each applicant:

- Consent statement from applicant to verify information and documents.
- Curriculum vitae, that includes education, training, and employment history.
- Confirmation from National Practitioner Data Bank (NPDB) and American Medical Association that applicant's information is accurate.
- Drug Enforcement Agency (DEA) Certificate.
- Copy of State License.
- Board Certificate(s) or Eligibility Letter(s).
- Statement regarding physical and mental health status in terms of his or her ability to perform requested privileges, including a statement regarding lack of impairment due to chemical dependency/substance abuse.
- Professional liability insurance for the past 5 years. Limits must be at least $1,000,000 per claim and $3,000,000 aggregate.
- Any and all involvement with professional liability action(s), including final judgments, settlement(s) or case(s) pending.
- Any and all past or pending professional disciplinary action(s), sanction(s), licensure limitation(s), or related matter(s).
- Termination(s) of medical staff membership; any and all voluntary or involuntary terminations.
- Any and all voluntary or involuntary limitation(s), reduction(s), or loss of clinical privileges at another institution.
- Three professional recommendations from peers.
- An attestation to the correctness/completeness of the Credentialing Application, state licenses, state controlled substance certificates, DEAs, malpractice facesheets, and board certification documents.
- A conflict of interest statement.
- Delineated privilege list.
- A signed statement agreeing to notify Quincy of any malpractice claims or changes in health status, and so forth that occur after completion of the application.

Sarah calls a meeting with all Quincy department directors. She explains that Quincy is hoping to create a database on LIPs that contains information that can be used in appointment/reappointment, privileging, marketing, contracting, performance measurement, and other activities. She writes two questions on the blackboard:

- If you could have any information on LIPs that provide care to Quincy's members, what would you ask for?
- Looking five years down the road, what information do you anticipate needing on LIPs who provide care to Quincy's members?

This meeting generates a long wish list of information that department directors would like on LIPs, including languages they spoke, hours of operation, e-mail addresses and fax numbers, research published, and boards they serve on.

Sally and Sarah also interview benefit managers at several employers that Quincy contracts with to learn what information they would like on providers. The customers are primarily interested in the quality and cost of care provided by various providers. In addition, several employers say they want to know what a provider's "philosophy of care" is (for example, did they emphasize wellness and prevention, holistic medicine).

Sally and Sarah take the "wish lists" obtained from talking to internal and external customers and determine what information can realistically be obtained on an application form. For example, a lot of performance information on LIPs (for example, patient outcomes) must be collected once they are appointed.

Sally and Sarah develop a draft application for LIPs to fill out when applying for appointment. They use example applications from other HMOs across the country, to create a draft application.

The team reviews and edits the draft application and runs it by the legal department to ensure it meets all laws and regulations. In addition, Phyllis suggests that Sally ask several LIPs at Quincy to fill out the application to see if it makes sense and is user-friendly. After Sally does this, she learns that several of the questions are confusing to LIPs and she makes the appropriate changes.

Identifying the appropriate software program. While Sally and Sarah are developing the appointment application, Doug Baron is researching and obtaining information on software applications that will help automate the credentialing and privileging process. After talking to vendors and other HMOs, he identifies eight possible programs that might fit the bill.

At a team meeting, he asks the members to help him identify criteria with which to rate the software applications. They decide on the following criteria:

- Customizes the screen to fit the application;
- Simplifies the paper-burden verification process;
- Creates a database of information on all LIPs;
- Operates over a network system and integrates with other organizational information systems;
- Fits within budget parameters; and
- Provides appropriate levels of security to prevent unauthorized access to confidential information.

After comparing the eight possible applications against criteria, Doug asks three software vendors to come in and demonstrate their packages. The team decides on one software application.

Identifying performance measures. Over the next several months, the team gradually completes the other tasks that need to be accomplished. One of the last tasks is to identify performance measures that will help them track the success of the newly designed credentialing system.

See page 69 for a discussion on indicators.

After much discussion, the team identifies three performance measures:

- 100% of LIPs are credentialed according to the criteria outlined in policies and procedures by January 1997;
- Mechanisms are in place to begin measuring and incorporating performance improvement information (for example, utilization information, patient outcomes, compliance with clinical guidelines) into the reappointment of physicians; and
- The credentialing process remains within budget parameters.

Piloting the Process

By July 1996, the task force is ready to pilot the new credentialing process. They decide to begin by appointing current members of their provider panel as well as all new applicants. They ask 25 members of the current provider panel to fill out applications each week as well as new applicants that ask to join Quincy. After the first month, the team will assess the process to see if any changes need to be made. The team hopes to have all current members appointed under the new system within six months. At that point, the team will assess the system against the established performance measures and make any necessary improvements.

Example 2-3. Developing a Hypertension Assessment Guideline

The Setting and Background

Located in a small eastern city, McHenry Hospital is a hypothetical 350-bed hospital that owns and manages two primary care clinics. One clinic is located next to the hospital; the other is located on the other side of the city. Hospital leaders have identified "the improvement of clinical outcomes and costs" as one of its strategic goals for the next two years. They intend to accomplish this goal primarily through developing and implementing clinical guidelines that help physicians manage disease processes.

Early in 1997, leaders ask the medical staff committee to develop and implement guidelines for five disease processes in the next year. Lead by the hospital's quality improvement director, committee members brainstorm a list of more than 30 possible processes on which to focus.

Example Highlights

Setting:
McHenry Hospital, Anycity, MA

Performance Improvement Initiatives:
Develop and implement a clinical guideline for hypertension assessment.

Dimensions of Performance Addressed:
Appropriateness, availability, continuity, effectiveness, efficacy, timeliness.

Comments:
This example illustrates how a team adapted a national guideline and identified performance measures to track the guideline's implementation.

To narrow the list, they compare the identified processes against four criteria:

- High volume;
- High risk;
- Problem prone; and
- Easily managed by a guideline.

Five processes, including hypertension assessment, meet all four criteria.

Design Process

Organizing a team. For each guideline, the director and his or her staff will convene a team of relevant caregivers. This development team will complete the up-front research and develop a draft guideline. The team will then present this draft guideline along with supporting evidence to the medical staff and other physician leaders for their approval.

To develop the hypertension guideline, the quality improvement director organizes a team of seven people from the hospital and its primary care clinics: two nurses, a physician assistant, a primary care physician, a dietician, a pharmacist, and a patient educator. In addition, a hypertension specialist is asked to serve as a consultant to the team.

Defining the process. The quality improvement director asks the team to draw a flowchart of the typical assessment of a patient with hypertension.

See page 104 for a discussion on flowcharts.

Team members are then asked to conduct outside research through literature review and telephone interviews with several clinics across the country with comparable patient populations to learn how they handle hypertension assessment.

From this research, the team learns that the detection rate for hypertension at the McHenry clinics is 15% lower than primary clinics with similar patient populations. Clinics with high detection rates follow one important practice—a standardized blood pressure measurement technique.

Adapting a national guideline. Rather than spending months developing a guideline on its own, the quality improvement director recommends that the team build on national and regional guidelines that have been published and disseminated. Team members review several such guidelines and select a hypertension guideline published by the National Heart, Lung, and Blood Institute.

The team revises the guideline to reflect practice in the McHenry clinics. The quality improvement director then presents this guideline to the hospital's medical staff committee and shows it to all primary care physicians and hypertension specialists connected with McHenry clinics. After the first review, the team incorporates the physicians' changes into the guideline and then asks them to review it a second time.

Collecting data on current process. The quality improvement director recommends that the team identify performance measures that will help them track whether the guideline is successfully implemented. To do this, the team identifies four critical junctures in the process and develops correlating measures:

See page 69 for a discussion on indicators.

- The percentage of patients who have their blood pressure checked at every office visit;
- The percentage of office visits in which staff correctly follow the standardized blood pressure measurement technique;
- The percentage of patients with consistent readings (that is, two or more readings taken on two or more separate occasions) of 140 mm Hg systolic and/or 90 mm Hg diastolic or higher who receive education and counseling on controlling high blood pressure; and
- All patients who are suspected of having secondary hypertension or resistant hypertension are referred to a hypertension specialist.

To obtain some baseline comparison data before piloting the guideline, the team decides to collect data on these measures for two weeks at one McHenry clinic. From this data collection, they find that many patients (21%) did not have their blood pressure measured during their office visit. As suspected, nurses used various blood pressure measurement techniques. Also, a large number of patients diagnosed with hypertension (22%) did not receive adequate education and counseling. The team was not able to obtain useful data on the last measure since only one patient was diagnosed with secondary or resistant hypertension during the two-week period.

Implementing the Guideline

The team decides to pilot the guideline at one primary care clinic first. Two nurses and a physician at that clinic have been put in charge of implementing the guideline. This implementation team plans to use the baseline data that was gathered to convince staff of the need for a standardized process for hypertension assessment. They are currently developing educational materials for a clinic in-service and putting processes in place that will help staff follow the guideline. At the same time, they collect baseline data on the clinic's current detection rate for hypertension as well as other performance data. After the guideline is implemented, they will collect data in approximately six months to learn how well they are complying with the guideline's recommendations and make any needed changes in practice. Then the implementation team will share what they have learned with staff at McHenry's other clinic and help them develop an appropriate implementation plan.

CHAPTER 3: Measure

Chapter Highlights

Why Do We Measure?

- To gain information about performance on an ongoing basis;
- To gain detailed information about a process chosen for assessment and improvement;
- To determine the effects of improvement actions; and
- To produce organization-specific performance databases.

What Do We Measure?

- Selected high-volume, high-risk, problem-prone, or costly processes on an ongoing basis;
- Selected processes, as indicated by ongoing measurement or other feedback;
- Customer experience and satisfaction; and
- Cross-functional, cross-discipline processes.

Who Performs the Measurement?

- Leaders with input from many sources (for example, staff, consumers, governance) decide what to measure on an ongoing basis;
- Organization staff trained in measurement techniques can help design ongoing measurement activities;

Continued on page 58.

Continued from page 57.

- Staff or consultants with expertise in information management should be involved in data collection, when possible; and
- Work groups or other teams measure processes chosen for intensive assessment and improvement.

Indicators

- An indicator is a valid and reliable quantitative measure related to one or more dimension of performance;
- Indicators can identify sentinel events or can show aggregate performance;
- Two types of aggregate-data indicators are rate-based and continuous-variable indicators; and
- Indicators can measure processes and outcome.

One Product of Measurement is a Performance Database

- The database provides aggregate information about process performance, outcomes, satisfaction, cost, and judgments about quality.

Examples of Performance Measurement

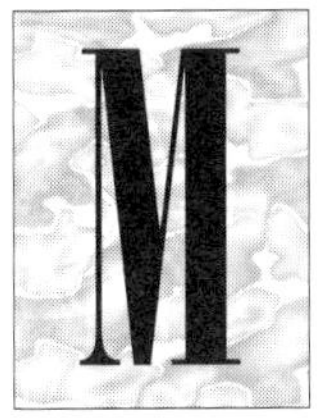

easurement is essential to improving the quality of ambulatory care. Performance measures can help focus improvement efforts and provide tools to judge the effectiveness of treatments, procedures, and other aspects of care. Measurement provides data that objectively describe how various functions or processes (for example, treatment of asthma patients, staff competency, infection control, and anesthesia use) are operating and what the outputs are.

In today's environment, accountability is also a pressing concern. Patients, payers, and others are demanding that health systems publicly report their performance in various areas. Every recent health care reform proposal includes requirements for measuring performance. Ambulatory care organizations must consistently and empirically demonstrate that their care meets performance standards and must measure patient outcomes, satisfaction, and costs.

Performance measurement is by no means unfamiliar in health care. Ambulatory care organizations routinely measure such indicators as the number of patients served, patient response to treatments, and staffing levels. However, for these measures to be meaningful, they must be tied into the organization's overall performance improvement efforts. Measurement is meaningless if the data simply sit on the shelf.

This chapter discusses an overall rationale for measurement and how measurement works within the cycle for improving performance (see Figure 3-1, page 60). This chapter answers the following questions:

- Why do we measure?
- What do we measure?
- Who performs the measurement?
- How do we measure?

Also included in this chapter are specific examples of how ambulatory care organizations can measure their performance. This information will guide organizations in achieving one important result of measurement: a performance database that can be used for tracking performance, establishing baseline data, and judging outcomes.

Why Do We Measure?

Chapter 2 described how to design a function or process. This is often the step where the improvement cycle begins. Measurement quickly follows design.

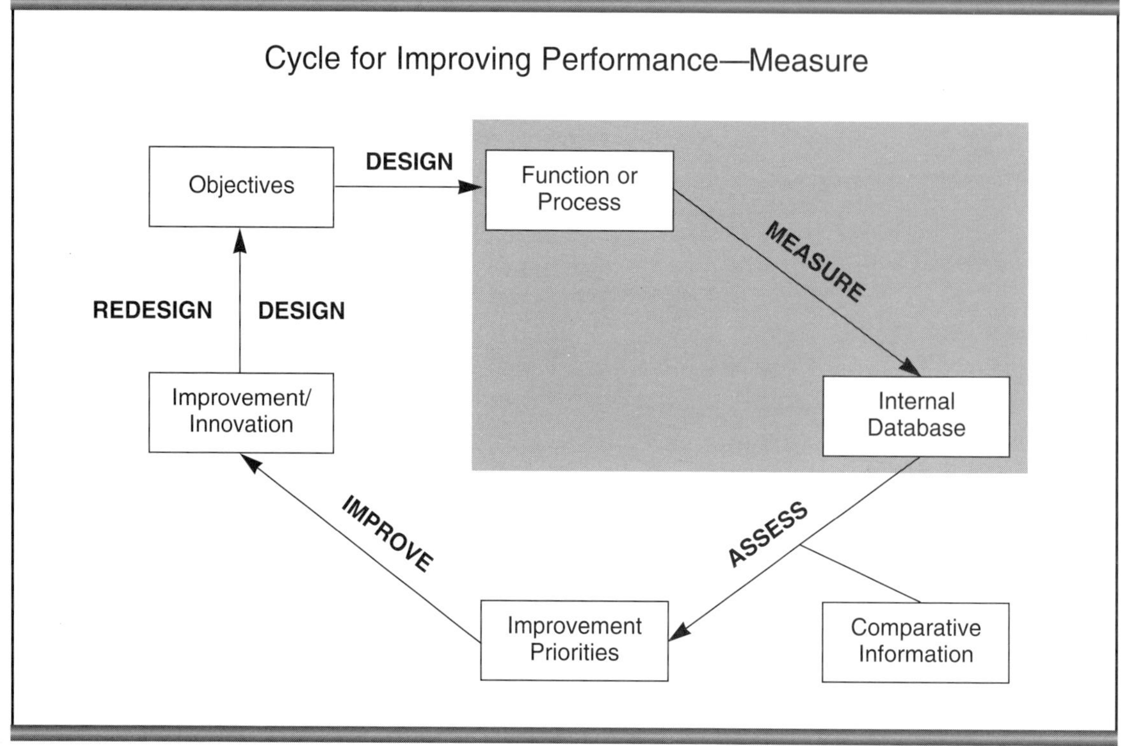

Figure 3-1. This figure highlights the measure stage of the improvement cycle.

When a new process is developed or an existing process is redesigned, an ambulatory care organization collects and aggregates data to learn how well the process performs. These data then help staff determine whether an improvement has occurred and whether additional improvement actions are necessary.

Measurement serves several purposes. One is to provide baseline data. This is particularly important when little objective information exists about a process. For example, organization leaders may want to learn whether staff are satisfied with various aspects of their work environment or staff may want to know the effectiveness of a new diabetic treatment program.

Staff can identify and collect data on specific indicators to learn more about a particular outcome or a particular step in a process. Once assessed, these data can help staff determine whether a process needs to be improved, and then they can begin a more intensive analysis. Data about costs and benefits, including costs of faulty or ineffective processes, may also be of significant interest to organization leaders and can be a vital part of ongoing performance measurement.

A second purpose of measurement is to gain more information about a process that was chosen for assessment and improvement. Consider the following findings:

- A target performance rate is not met (for example, a drug complication rate is too high or a patient satisfaction indicator is too low);
- A performance rate varies significantly from the previous year, from day to day, or from the statistical average (for example, the average time to respond to laboratory orders increases or wait time for new patient appointments increases); or
- Patient or staff feedback indicates dissatisfaction with performance (for example, the number of complaints from patients about long waiting times increases or staff express concerns about inadequate phone lines).

Each of these findings may cause an ambulatory care organization to focus on a given process and determine opportunities for improvement. Detailed measurement would then be necessary to gather additional data about exactly how the process performs and about factors affecting that performance.

Finally, measurement helps to determine the effectiveness of improvement actions. Once a process is changed or modified, staff must monitor the effect that change has on future performance. For example, if an imaging facility institutes a new process for transferring patient records to other providers, then staff would first need to establish how well the current process meets certain performance measures (that is, determine the baseline rate) and then continue measuring those indicators after adopting the new process.

Measurement can also be used to demonstrate that key processes (for example, the preparation, delivery, and administration of medications) are "in control." Understanding variation over time and whether a process is, in fact, in control (that is, within acceptable limits of variation) is vital for continuous process improvement. Once a process has been stabilized at an acceptable level of performance, measures may be taken periodically to verify that improvement has been sustained.

One important end result of measurement is an organization-specific performance database. Such databases are invaluable for organization improvement and may link information at multiple levels (for example, practitioner, program, patient, and organization) about process performance, outcomes, satisfaction, cost, and customer judgments.

Thus, measurement provides many benefits to organizations interested in continuously improving their performance. Several important benefits include:

- *Measurement creates a common language* that provides a degree of precision and clarity often needed to identify, analyze, and resolve important ambulatory health care issues.
- *Measurement establishes benchmarks,* or points of reference, for performance. Benchmarks are used by organizations to identify potential opportunities for improvement and to determine whether performance has in fact improved and by how much. Benchmarks are increasingly being used by ambulatory care organizations, users, and payers of services to determine whether their expectations for performance have been met.
- *Measurements provide organizations with data* that can be used to set performance improvement priorities.
- *Measurement improves the accuracy* with which ambulatory care professionals observe, record, and form conclusions through data analysis about important processes and functions.
- *Measurement keeps health care professionals clearly focused* on real improvement opportunities.
- *Measurement fosters participants' acceptance of, and involvement in,* the goals and processes of performance improvement activities.
- *Measurement provides milestones* toward which people can strive.

What Do We Measure? Setting Priorities

An ambulatory care organization cannot and should not measure everything simultaneously. Its activities are too diverse and its resources too limited. Therefore, the organization's leaders, in concert with staff, must find the most productive way to measure vital or important processes. One method is to measure certain outcomes or aspects of a process that can potentially identify larger performance issues.

The topic, "what do we measure," is also related to what an ambulatory care organization defines as its work and prime deliverables. For example, a student health service might track the reasons students access the system. Or an endoscopy center might measure costs and patient outcomes for key diagnostic procedures. When performance rates in important areas show significant variation or do not achieve targets, a more detailed measurement and assessment should be initiated.

Leaders need to determine which processes will be subject to ongoing measurement. They must carefully weigh the processes' relationships to the organization's mission, vision, and resources. In addition, the concerns, needs, and preferences of the provider, individual being served, family, community, purchaser, physician, referral source, and payer must be considered.

Table 3-1, below, depicts one possible method for identifying important processes to measure, assess, and improve. Using this methodology, an ambulatory care center periodically surveys its patients, physicians, employees, and payers to help identify priorities for process measurement and improvement within the organization. In this example, a primary care center developed a crosswalk to highlight potential processes to evaluate. They listed key customers, Joint Commission's functions, the organization's important clinical services, and the Joint Commission's nine dimensions of performance. In this way, they decided to focus on effectiveness of assessing diabetic patients.

Table 3-1. Example Methodology for Identifying Important Processes to Measure, Assess, and Improve

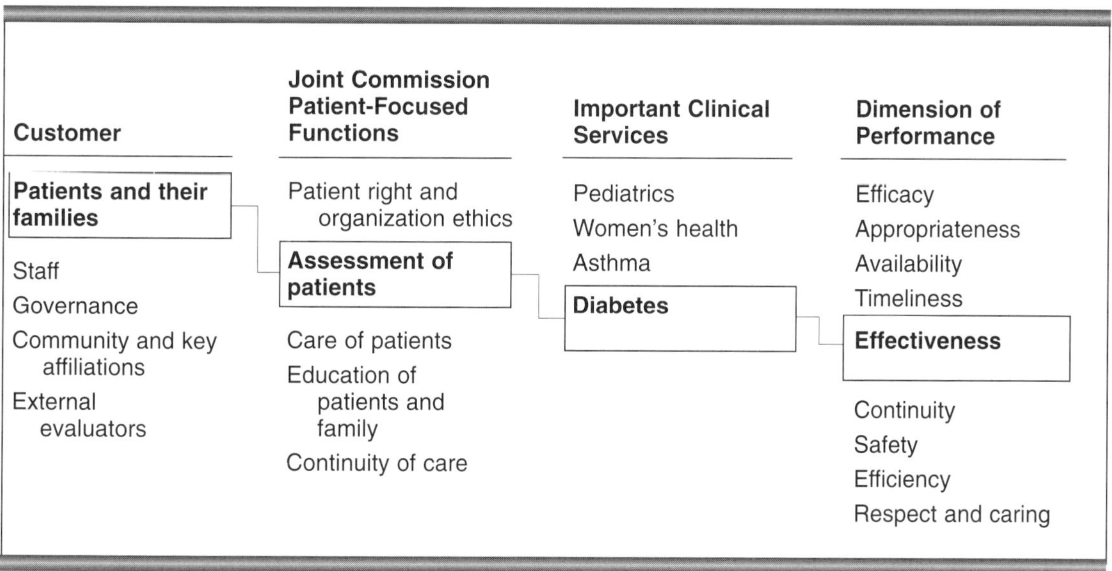

Customer	Joint Commission Patient-Focused Functions	Important Clinical Services	Dimension of Performance
Patients and their families	Patient right and organization ethics	Pediatrics	Efficacy
Staff	**Assessment of patients**	Women's health	Appropriateness
Governance	Care of patients	Asthma	Availability
Community and key affiliations	Education of patients and family	**Diabetes**	Timeliness
External evaluators	Continuity of care		**Effectiveness**
			Continuity
			Safety
			Efficiency
			Respect and caring

Other important factors to consider when choosing processes to continuously measure include standards or requirements from regulating or accrediting bodies, including the Joint Commission. For example, the Joint Commission identifies a number of important functions that may be the subject of ongoing measurement as listed in Table 3-2, below. This list of functions is worth considering because it provides one frame of reference for an ambulatory care organization that is conceptualizing its measurement activities. Measurement activities can also be organized around patient diagnoses, critical paths, product and service lines, or other factors. The Joint Commission's functions are broad and the associated standards intentionally allow considerable flexibility for measurement within each function.

Within these functions, specific processes or outcomes may be selected for measurement. The processes or outcomes typically chosen will

- affect a large percentage of clients, or are high volume (for example, Pap smears at a women's clinic);
- place individuals at serious risk if not performed well, performed when not indicated, or not performed when indicated, or are high risk (for example, IV site infections);

Table 3-2. Important Functions to Consider for Ongoing Measurement

Patient-Focused Functions

- Patient rights and organization ethics
- Assessment of patients
- Care of patients
- Patient education
- Continuity of care

Organization Functions

- Improving organization performance
- Leadership
- Management of the environment of care
- Management of human resources
- Management of information
- Surveillance, prevention, and control of infection

- have been or are likely to be associated with problems, or are problem prone (for example, clinic waiting times);
- be costly (for example, drug selection); or
- represent cross-organization functions (for example, staff competency).

The Joint Commission's standards also identify some important sources of data for measuring performance that an ambulatory care organization should consider:

- Staff, patients served, and others' views about the organization's performance, perceived problems, and opportunities for improvement;
- Risk management activities; and
- Quality control activities, including clinical laboratory services.

Patient Satisfaction and Experience

Ambulatory care organizations should measure patient satisfaction and experience with all aspects of care. Crosswalking a patient's experience with the dimensions of performance, and integrating this information with organization-wide efforts will likely improve performance with traditional components of patient satisfaction:

- Personal aspects of care;
- Technical quality of care;
- Accessibility and availability of care;
- Continuity of care;
- Convenience to the individual served;
- Physical setting;
- Financial considerations; and
- Efficacy of treatment.

Feedback from patients served, families, physicians, referral sources, and staff can help an organization determine what processes need attention or identify a process's weaknesses and strengths.

Who Performs the Measurement?

The staff responsible for performing measurement activities will differ depending on the goals and nature of the measurement undertaken. Two important ideas helpful when conducting measurement activities include: 1) tailoring and superimposing measurement activities into existing, ongoing data collection activities; and 2) conducting measurement activities as close in time to the occurrence of the measurement events as possible. The following sections provide some general guidelines on who may be responsible for and involved in designing and collecting data for measurement.

Staff Involved in Ongoing Measurement to Monitor a Process

Some ambulatory care organizations are fortunate to have various experts who can help design measurement activities, including information management, quality improvement, and the specific functions to be measured. Other organizations without in-house expertise will self-educate, form strategic alliances with other groups, or import these talents from elsewhere. At a minimum, the organization's leaders must review and approve the design of measurement activities.

The people involved will vary widely depending on the specific organization, on the process being measured, and on the measurement process itself. As noted earlier, organizations should make every effort to coordinate ongoing measurement with data collection already taking place as part of everyday activities. In addition, organizations should develop comprehensive data dictionaries that define the data elements, recording cycles, and owners of the processes. These dictionaries help the organization's staff keep track of what is being measured and forces them to carefully plan and define the measurement activities.

Staff Involved in Measurement for a Specific Improvement Effort

Measurement for a specific improvement effort is typically more detailed than routine screening. When an organization has decided to improve a particular process (for example, reporting of adverse drug reactions or patient education about medication side effects), it can empower a specific group to study the process, and recommend and implement changes. This group could be an existing team or a special team composed of those involved in the process being studied. It will usually be responsible for designing and carrying out the measurement activities necessary to determine how the process performs. After making changes to improve the process, the team should continue to apply some or all of its measures to determine whether the change has had the desired effect.

How Do We Measure?

Ambulatory care organizations carry out several basic types of measurement:

- Ongoing measurement of selected outcomes or aspects of the process that most powerfully influence the outcome (related to quality control);
- Measurement of priority issues chosen for improvement (part of a more intensive assessment and improvement effort, which may be initiated based on the results of ongoing measurement and performance data); and
- Measures collected for one purpose that can be used to examine another process or function (secondary analysis approach); a practical method to collect important data without generating a new data-gathering effort.

The measurement and analysis of any data may provide insight into multiple processes. To carry out all three types of measurements, an organization needs to establish indicators or performance measures.

Indicators

An indicator is a valid and reliable quantitative process or outcomes measure related to one or more of the dimensions of performance described in Chapter 1 (efficacy, appropriateness, availability, timeliness, effectiveness, continuity, safety, efficiency, and respect and caring). As summarized in Table 3-3, below, an indicator has the following key characteristics:

- *Quantitative.* Quantitative data represent information expressed in specific measurement units. These data do not alone express any judgment or conclusion about the process being measured. They provide specific, objective information requiring further study, analysis, and interpretation.

Table 3-3. Indicator Defined

An indicator is

- **Quantitative**—expressed in units of measurement.
- **Valid**—identifies events that merit review.
- **Reliable**—accurately and completely identifies occurrences.
- **A measure of process**—a goal-directed series of activities or **outcome**—the results of performance.

- ***Valid.*** An indicator is considered valid if the measurement correctly captures the event of interest, identifies an opportunity for improving performance, or identifies a phenomenon that merits further review, which is a step toward identifying an improvement opportunity.
- ***Reliable.*** An indicator is considered reliable if it yields the same estimate by the same observer on multiple occasions or when it yields the same estimate by multiple observers of the same event. Reliability estimates confirm that the same measurement has consistently been obtained for the same event.
- ***Identifies a specific element of the process being measured or an outcome of that process.*** Outcomes measurement is necessary to learn results from improvement efforts and may record existing levels of and changes in health status, knowledge or behavior relevant to future health status, and satisfaction and experience with health care personnel. Process measurement is designed to identify what caused those results.

In any health care organization, the relationship between process and outcomes is complex. Hence, outcomes do not directly assess quality of performance but rather permit an inference about the process of care. Also, because the outcomes of many clinical processes may not be evident or measurable at the time of specific events (for example, end of clinic visit or discharge from a surgery center) or may vary considerably due to patient-specific factors, it is prudent to measure the processes that most profoundly influence the anticipated outcome and the outcome itself.

An example of an outcomes indicator is "patients with cardiac disease who demonstrate a reversal in coronary blockage and decrease in chest pain." A process indicator might be "cardiac patients receive proper education about nutrition and exercise." An outcomes indicator for environmental and life safety services might be "the number of staff who can correctly perform a fire drill procedure on request."

For your convenience, "Appendix A: Indicators for Ambulatory Care" contains an excerpt from the *National Library of Healthcare Indicators™ (NLHI™): Health Plan and Network Edition,* a new Joint Commission publication containing 225 indicator profiles. These indicators have passed a face-validity screening process, but are not necessarily endorsed by the Joint Commission.

Types of Indicators

Two types of indicators are sentinel-event indicators and aggregate-data indicators. A *sentinel-event indicator* identifies an individual event or occurrence that is significant and defined to trigger further review, study, and investigation each time it occurs. Most sentinel events are highly undesirable and occur infrequently. The following are several examples of sentinel events in an ambulatory care setting:

- A patient complaint of negligent staff;
- Medication error or allergic reaction to drug; or
- Patient requiring transfer to higher level of care (for example, hospital admission after outpatient surgery or unscheduled hospital admission within 72 hours of clinic visit).

Such indicators are well known in risk management. In quality management systems, they help ensure that each adverse event is promptly evaluated to prevent future occurrences.

Although sentinel-event indicators are useful to help ensure some basic functions (for example, patient safety), they are less useful in measuring the overall level of performance in an organization. This is particularly true when they are the only indicators of organization performance. In part, this is true because of the rare occurrence of these events, and also because they often represent special, as opposed to common-cause, variation in organizations. A specific-cause or special-cause variation represents a unique set of circumstances not regularly present in the system. To mount a quality improvement effort based on special-cause variation would be a mistake.

In contrast, an *aggregate-data indicator* quantifies a process or outcome that may be related to many causes. Unlike sentinel events, an event identified by an aggregate-data indicator may occur frequently. For example, a primary care clinic may want to monitor the care given to asthmatic patients. To do so, they might measure the number of asthmatic children admitted to the hospital each month. A hospital admission for an asthmatic child is serious, and the patient's physician should assess the reason (for example, the child is not using inhaler correctly) and provide appropriate follow-up care. However, this event does not warrant a clinicwide investigation each time it occurs. On the other hand, if the number of asthmatic children admitted to the hospital exceeds acceptable proportions, as predetermined by clinic staff, then staff should investigate whether overall process or system causes are to blame (for example, asthmatic children are not being effectively taught how to use their inhalers).

Aggregate-data indicators are divided into two groups: rate-based indicators and continuous-variable indicators.

Rate-based indicators. Rate-based indicators express information in proportions or ratios. Typically, the proportion of the number of occurrences to the entire group within which the occurrence could take place are shown, as in the following examples:

$$\frac{\text{patients with diabetes who require foot amputation}}{\text{all individuals with diabetes}}$$

$$\frac{\text{number of no-show appointments}}{\text{total patient visits}}$$

$$\frac{\text{women receiving mammograms who require treatment}}{\text{women who receive mammograms}}$$

The rate can also express a ratio comparing the occurrences identified with a different, but related, phenomenon. For example,

$$\frac{\text{patients with fasting blood sugar greater than 160 mg}}{\text{total patient visits for diabetes}}$$

Continuous-variable indicators. This type of aggregate-data indicator measures performance along a continuous scale. For example, a continuous-variable indicator might track the number of immunizations completed or record the number of patient visits. Whereas a rate-based indicator might express the proportion of the delivery responses that are greater than two hours to the total delivery responses, a continuous-variable indicator would measure the specific delivery response time, thus offering more precise information.

Staff who design measurement activities must consider the process being measured, the goals of measurement, and the available data so as to choose the best

Table 3-4. Types of Indicators

Aggregate data indicator: A performance measure based on collection and aggregation of data about many events or phenomena. The events or phenomena may be desirable or undesirable, and the data may be reported as a continuous variable or as a discrete variable (or rate).

Continuous variable indicator: An aggregate data indicator in which the value of each measurement can fall anywhere along a continuous scale (for example, the number of immunizations)

Rate-based (or discrete variable) indicator: An aggregate data indicator in which the value of each measurement is expressed as a proportion or as a ratio. In a proportion, the numerator is expressed as a subset of the denominator (for example, children who receive immunizations versus all children in patient population). In a ratio, the numerator and denominator measure different phenomena (for example, the number of patients with symptoms of depression versus the number of disability days attributable to depression).

Sentinel event indicator: A performance measure that identifies an individual event or phenomenon that always triggers further analysis and investigation; it usually occurs infrequently and is undesirable in nature (for example, patient adverse incidents).

type or types of indicators. Table 3-4, above, summarizes the different types of indicators; the examples in this chapter provide illustrations of how indicators are used to measure performance.

Using Indicators

When selecting or developing a measurement system, staff should consider several important concepts to ensure balance. First, consider different types of measures to illuminate various aspects of the process (for example, measures of process and outcome, sentinel-event and aggregate-data indicators). Second, the appropriate dimensions of performance should be considered and indicators should be tailored to address them. No single dimension eclipses the others; all are essential for an organization pursuing excellence in performance.

Figure 3-2, page 72, illustrates the relationships among important functions, patient populations, and dimensions of performance. Any of these factors may provide the impetus for measurement and serve as a gateway to the framework for improving performance. After determining what measures will be most useful, an organization could then examine the linkages between the patient population, dimensions of performance, and important functions. For example, a group practice measuring care provided to patients with congestive heart failure might focus on the appropriateness or efficacy (a dimension of performance) of patient education (an important function).

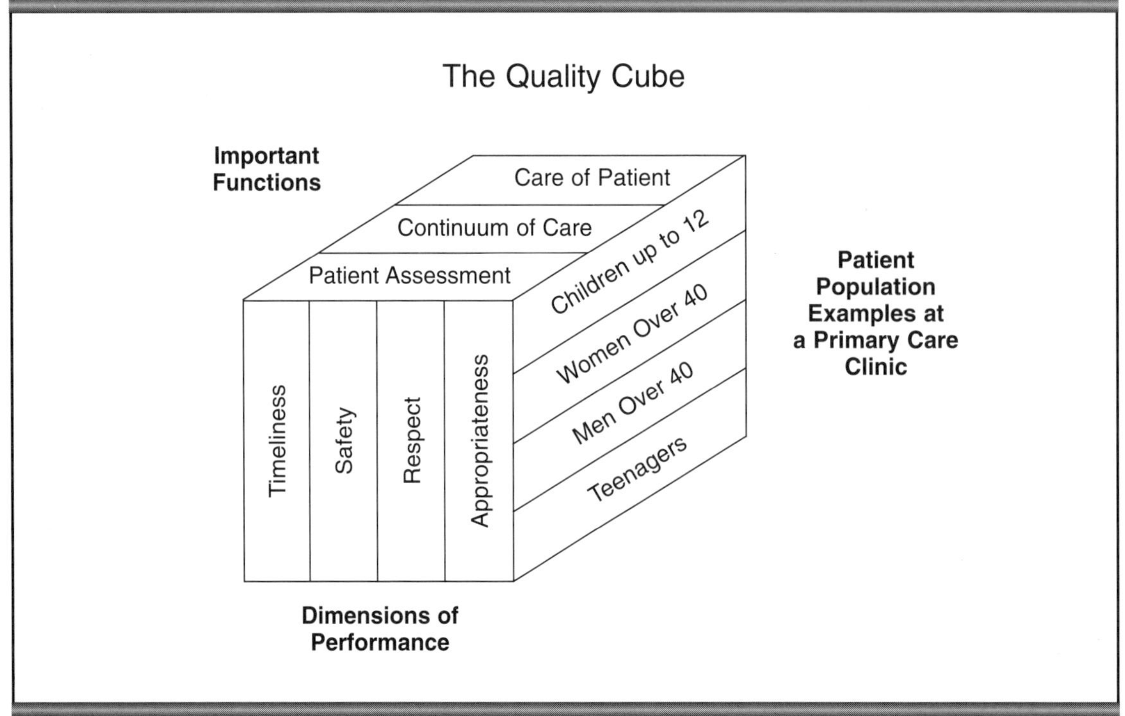

Figure 3-2. This figure illustrates the relationships among some dimensions of performance, some important functions, and some patient population types for a primary care clinic.

Examples of Performance Measurement

The following examples are designed to provide a range of approaches to ongoing measurement; no one approach is the best for every organization, and none are specifically required by Joint Commission standards. The examples are adapted from actual practices and represent common problems or challenges faced by ambulatory care organizations. These examples illustrate how organizations evaluate ambulatory care structures, collect information about how a particular process is performing, and measure critical outcomes.

Example 3-1. Measuring Drug Prescription Patterns at a University-Based Health Clinic

The Setting and Background

The medical department at the Massachusetts Institute of Technology (MIT) in Cambridge is a university-based health clinic that provides care to a patient population of approximately 25,000 people. The department serves the MIT student population, faculty, and staff through a staff-model HMO, which began in 1973 as one of the Boston area's first HMOs.

Example Highlights

Setting:
Massachusetts Institute of Technology, University Health Clinic, Cambridge, Massachussetts

Performance Improvement Initiative:
Reduce drug costs while ensuring effective treatment.

Dimensions of Performance Addressed:
Appropriateness, availability, continuity, effectiveness, efficiency.

Comments:
This example illustrates how an educative team approach reduces drug costs, ensures quality of care, and maintains physician satisfaction.

The Problem

During the 1994 budget process, it became obvious that MIT's drug costs were steadily increasing. The total cost of drugs used in filling prescriptions more than doubled in five years, growing from $662,015 in 1988 to $1,444,261 in 1993. Concerned, clinic leaders asked a team of people to look into why these costs were increasing and to see if they could identify potential areas for cost savings.

For several months, the assistant medical director, senior manager for operations, and pharmacy director met to review data on drug costs. They consulted with the laboratory director, medical director, and the chairperson of the Pharmacy and Therapeutics Committee. The team examined the number of prescriptions filled in relation to enrollment, the inflation rate, and new drug products. The goal was to ascertain what costs could be controlled and what costs were beyond control.

The results showed that inflation was responsible for an increase in drug costs, accounting for 47% of the increase, and growth in membership accounted for another 8% (see Figure 3-3, page 74). However, 45% of the increase in drug costs was attributable to physician choice—that is, the drugs physicians chose to prescribe.

The team identified two factors related to physician prescribing patterns that contributed to the escalation in drug costs:

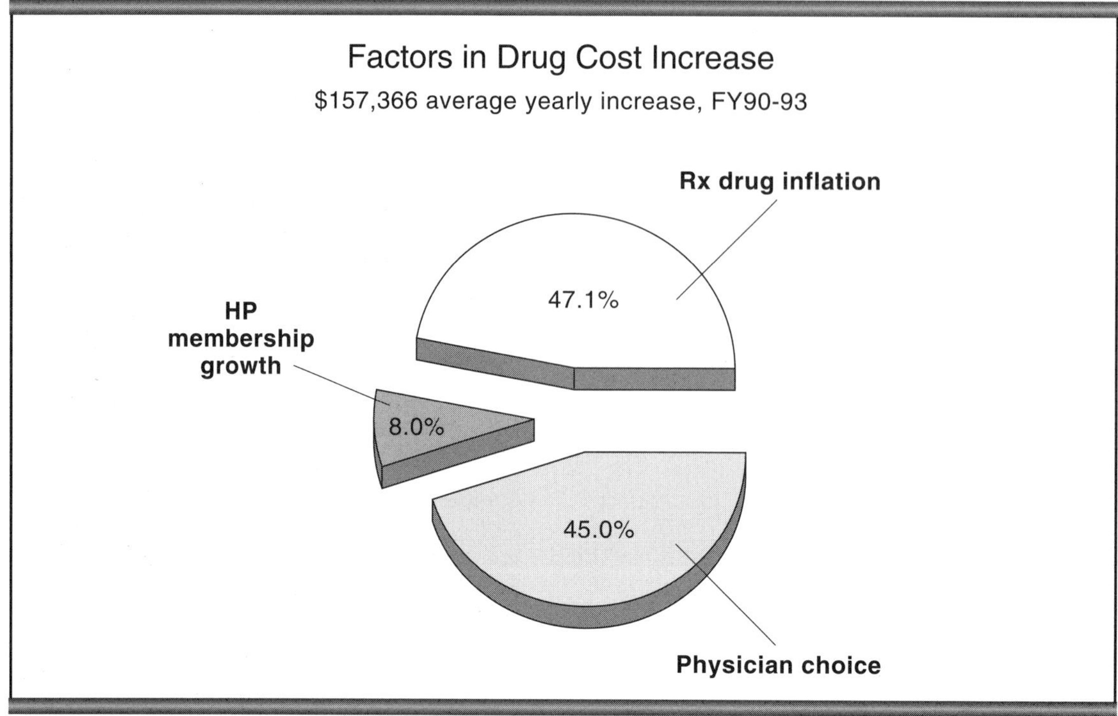

Figure 3-3. After reviewing data on drug costs, staff found that 45% of the increase in drug costs from 1988 to 1993 was attributable to physician choice—that is, the drugs physicians chose to prescribe.
Source: **Massachusetts Institute of Technology, Cambridge, MA. Used with permission.**

- Utilization rate per member. The number of medications prescribed to each patient had risen steadily. In the past five years, the average number of prescriptions per health plan member per year had increased by 46%, from 3.6 per member per year in 1988 to 5.27 per member per year in 1993.
- Product mix. Sophisticated technology, preferred "new-and-improved" products, and expensive brand name products were driving up drug costs.

Team members felt that the department could cut costs, without sacrificing quality, by educating and encouraging physicians to prescribe less expensive products whenever appropriate.

Designing Solution

In the late 1980s, the pharmacy department had made some fledgling attempts to contain drug costs by focusing on specific high-cost drugs. The efforts were only minimally successful because physicians felt the focus was often on products that were not widely used.

The team looked for another approach. Having clinical and administrative members as well as representatives from ancillary services on the team allowed the group to carefully examine all aspects of their provider's prescribing patterns. Factors such as patient population and case mix could be evaluated along with clinical disease management.

Physicians needed information on drug costs and regular feedback about the prescribing patterns. With this in mind, the team felt that it would be more effective to focus on all aspects of management of a disease or condition (for example, depression, or hypertension), rather than to target a particular drug. Recommendations were established for treatment of the whole disease state and, when clinically equivalent, use of the least expensive drug was encouraged.

To help determine what conditions to focus on, the pharmacy established that the most expensive drugs used at MIT primarily fell into four treatment categories:

- Hypertension;
- Hypercholesterolemia;
- Gastrointestinal disorders; and
- Depression.

Any savings realized by more effective disease management and drug cost containment in these groups would, therefore, be significant (see Table 3-5, page 76, for the drug list).

Targeting Hypertension

The team decided to organize educational sessions for their first disease management category. They used an expert in the field to lead the meeting and present various drug therapies and their costs. Physicians were not required to use particular drugs but were given information necessary to make cost-effective decisions.

Following these meetings, each physician received quarterly reports that detailed his or her drug utilization by cost for antihypertensive drugs. Included in the report were charts that compared a physician's average daily medication cost per patient to that of his or her peers (see Figure 3-4, page 77).

Table 3-5. Most Expensive Drugs for 1993 and 1994

	Drug	Cost	
		1994 (Annualized)	1993
1	PROZAC 20 mg PULVULE	137,982	106,701
2	ZANTAC 150 mg TABLET	81,279	73,620
3	PERGONAL 75 IU AMPULE	65,004	36,546
4	MEVACOR 20 mg TABLET	59,886	47,956
5	ZOLOFT 100 mg TABLET	30,795	21,842
6	BETASERON 0.3 mg VIAL	29,682	N/A
7	VASOTEC 5 mg TABLET	25,401	25,542
8	METRODIN 75 IU AMPULE	24,741	15,697
9	PRILOSEC 20 mg CAPSULE SA	24,555	18,065
10	VASOTEC 10 mg TABLET	22,485	23,617
11	MEVACOR 40 mg TABLET	21,558	16,584
12	CALAN SR 240 mg CAPLET SA	21,474	22,538
13	RECOMBIVAX HB 10 mcg/ml VIAL	21,171	12,245
14	SELDANE 60 mg TABLET	21,126	30,326
15	PREMARIN 0.625 mg TABLET	19,941	16,010
16	KLONOPIN 0.5 mg TABLET	19,056	19,625
17	PROTROPIN 10 mg KIT W/DIL	18,900	14,700
18	CIPRO 500 mg TABLET	18,765	15,502
19	LUPRON DEPOT 3.75 mg KIT	18,687	6,383
20	NEUPOGEN 300 mcg/ml VIAL	17,490	9,199
21	SANDIMMUNE 100 mg CAPSULE	17,427	14,062
22	ACCUTANE 40 mg CAPSULE	17,304	8,369
23	ZOLADEX 3.6 mg IMPLANT SYRN	17,295	10,133
24	VASOTEC 20 mg TABLET	14,901	12,209
25	NOLVADEX 10 mg TABLET	13,956	14,424
26	PAXIL 20 mg TABLET	13,851	4,729
27	PROZAC 10 mg PULVULE	13,815	8,127
28	ZOVIRAX 200 mg CAPSULE	13,071	9,244
29	ONE TOUCH TEST STRIPS	11,925	9,799
30	TAGAMET 400 mg TABLET	11,511	10,751
31	KLONOPIN 1 mg TABLET	10,791	8,491
32	PROCARDIA XL 30 mg TABLET SA	10,662	12,135

Source: **Massachusetts Institute of Technology, Cambridge, MA. Used with permission.**

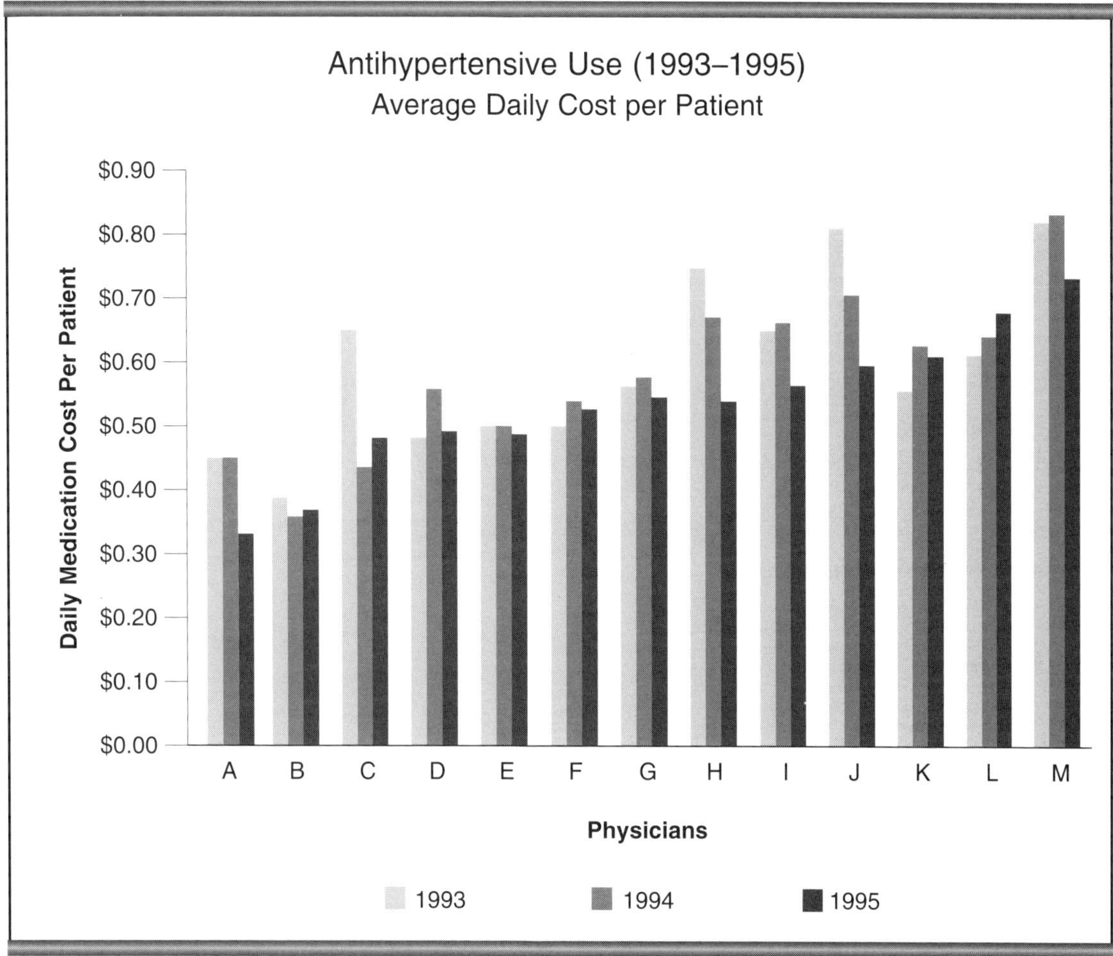

Figure 3-4. Physicians receive quarterly reports comparing their average daily medication cost per patient to that of their peers.
***Source:* Massachusetts Institute of Technology, Cambridge, MA. Used with permission.**

The chair of the Pharmacy and Therapeutics Committee received a copy of each physician report, enabling him to privately discuss prescribing patterns with physicians who were outside the norm.

See page 103 for a discussion on histograms.

To account for differences in patient mix, drug utilization costs were averaged. Each physician's average daily cost of medication per hypertension patient was calculated so that physicians seeing more hypertensive patients did not show higher costs. To calculate this, the costs of all drugs prescribed by a provider were divided by the number of patient days of medication dispensed.

Over the course of 1994, similar programs were implemented for three other treatment categories: depression, gastrointestinal disorders, and hypercholesterolemia. A similar process was followed, using external and internal expertise to educate physicians about drug costs and provide regular feedback about prescribing patterns.

A year after implementing the program, the pharmacy director met with each physician individually to discuss his or her drug costs and any specific questions. Through pharmacy newsletters, physicians received cost-containment information and reminders about recommended prescribing choices.

One year after implementing the cost containment program, drug costs were reduced by $75,000.

Next Steps

It was also important to verify that less costly drugs were as effective as more expensive drugs. Therapeutic quality should not be sacrificed in order to use a less costly product. In one study, the pharmacy examined LDL levels in patients receiving various drugs to see if they were adversely affected by switching drugs. They were not negatively affected.

Currently, the pharmacy is working with providers and other departments, such as health education, to educate patients about their conditions, the medications used, and any life-style changes that could benefit their care. In addition to patient-specific information, the pharmacy targets a different health issue each month.

Example 3-2. Measuring Physician Satisfaction at a Surgery Center

The Setting and Background

The Tallahassee Single Day Surgery Center has four operating rooms and 12 recovery beds. It is owned by a group of 43 surgeons and is not affiliated with a hospital or health system. The center performs 4,500 procedures a year in eight specialities: gynecology, urology, ENT, general surgery, ophthalmology, plastic surgery, podiatry, and orthopedics.

The surgery center has been using performance improvement concepts and principles since its inception. It views performance improvement as a tool to help provide high-quality, cost-effective outpatient elective surgical care.

Example Highlights

Setting:
Tallahassee Single Day Surgery Center, Tallahassee, Florida

Performance Improvement Initiative:
Monitor and improve physician satisfaction with the center's services and equipment.

Dimensions of Performance Addressed:
Availability, effectiveness, timeliness.

Comments:
This example illustrates how a data collection effort can be used to improve multiple areas of performance.

Identifying Customers

To compete for surgical cases with local hospitals and surgery centers, the center's board members realized that they had to please three customer groups: patients, payers, and physicians.

The surgery center was already measuring patient satisfaction on a regular basis. However, they did not have a good understanding of surgeons' perceptions. The executive director was asked to develop and implement a physician satisfaction survey. This survey was to

- pinpoint physicians' ratings of the surgery center compared to other centers;
- identify areas that could be improved; and
- validate what the organization was doing right.

Designing the Survey

The executive director decided to adapt a pre-existing survey and gave it to the other members of the Quality Improvement (QI) Committee to examine. The QI Committee decided to ask surgeons to rate surgical equipment and instruments (see Figure 3-5, page 80). At the time, the surgery center was considering replacing or refurbishing all the equipment and instruments in the center. The QI Committee decided to use this survey to determine which instruments and equipment surgeons felt needed updating.

Physician Satisfaction Survey

1. Please put an X next to your specialty.

❑ Dental	❑ Orthopedic
❑ ENT	❑ Pain Management
❑ General Surgery	❑ Plastic/Cosmetic
❑ Gastroenterology	❑ Podiatry
❑ Gynecology	❑ Urology
❑ Ophthalmology	❑ Other, please specify ______________________

2. How long have you been using our facility?
   - ❑ Less than 1 year
   - ❑ 1 to 3 years
   - ❑ 3 to 5 years
   - ❑ Over 5 years

3. How much do the following influence your decision to use the surgery center?

	Very Much	Somewhat	Not Much	Not at All
A. Insurance and HMO/PPOs	❑	❑	❑	❑
B. Prices for patient procedures	❑	❑	❑	❑
C. Quality of anesthesia	❑	❑	❑	❑
D. Quality/professionalism of staff	❑	❑	❑	❑
E. Efficient use of your time	❑	❑	❑	❑
F. Patient request	❑	❑	❑	❑
G. Availability of OR time	❑	❑	❑	❑

4. How would you rate the following:

	Excellent	Above Average	Average	Poor
A. Ease of scheduling	❑	❑	❑	❑
B. Equipment and instruments	❑	❑	❑	❑
C. Turnaround time	❑	❑	❑	❑
D. Promptness of surgery start time	❑	❑	❑	❑
E. Efficiency and knwledge of staff	❑	❑	❑	❑
F. Responsiveness to needs	❑	❑	❑	❑
G. Physical facilities	❑	❑	❑	❑
H. Care given to patients	❑	❑	❑	❑
I. Pre-op visits	❑	❑	❑	❑
J. Cost	❑	❑	❑	❑
K. Expedience of pathology reports	❑	❑	❑	❑
L. Amount of paperwork involved	❑	❑	❑	❑
M. Courtesy of front office staff	❑	❑	❑	❑
N. Patient satisfaction with billing office	❑	❑	❑	❑

5. How does the surgery center compare to other medical facilities you use?

	Better	About the Same	Worse
A. Ease of scheduling	❑	❑	❑
B. Equipment	❑	❑	❑
C. Turnaround time	❑	❑	❑
D. Surgery start time	❑	❑	❑
E. Efficiency and knowledge of staff	❑	❑	❑
F. Responsiveness to needs	❑	❑	❑
G. Physical facilities	❑	❑	❑
H. Care given to patients	❑	❑	❑
I. Pre-op visits	❑	❑	❑
J. Cost	❑	❑	❑
K. Expedience of pathology reports	❑	❑	❑
L. Amount of paperwork involved	❑	❑	❑
M. Courtesy of front office staff	❑	❑	❑
N. Patient satisfaction with billing office	❑	❑	❑

We would appreciate your comments and suggestions on how we can make our existing services better or what new services would be helpful to you.

____

____

____

Thank you for your cooperation.

Figure 3-5. The center took a physician satisfaction survey they found in the literature, added additional questions, and adapted it for their own purposes.
***Source:* Tallahassee Single Day Surgery Center, Tallahassee, FL. Used with permission.**

As a measurement goal, the QI Committee decided that "85% of surgeons will rate us better than other medical facilities on all survey items." If they did not achieve this threshold for any particular survey item, the QI Committee would conduct an in-depth improvement study in that area.

See page 69 for a discussion on indicators.

Baseline Survey Results

The survey was mailed to all 62 surgeons who used the surgery center in 1992. Thirty-seven surveys were returned for a response rate of 59.7%. For the most part, the findings were extremely positive. The QI Committee learned that the majority of surgeons rated the surgery center as excellent or above average in the following 14 characteristics (see Figure 3-6, page 82):

See page 107 for a discussion on Pareto charts.

- Ease of scheduling;
- Equipment and instruments;
- Turnaround time;
- Promptness of surgery start time;
- Efficiency and knowledge of staff;
- Responsiveness to needs;
- Physical facilities;
- Care given to patients;
- Preoperative visits;
- Cost;
- Expedience of pathology reports;
- Amount of paperwork involved;
- Courtesy of front office staff; and
- Patient satisfaction with billing.

The survey helped the QI Committee members pinpoint one area that needed improvement—promptness of surgery time. Twenty-two surgeons said Tallahassee Single Day Surgery was only average in this area compared to other medical centers.

In addition, the QI Committee was able to determine which surgical instruments needed refurbishing by breaking down the data into type of surgeons. From this data the committee members learned that many gynecologists rated the center's instruments and equipment below average.

Improvement Actions

To increase staff awareness of physician needs, the survey findings were presented and discussed at a staff meeting. At this time, surgery center staff also discussed the problem of surgery start times. The surgery center began initiatives to improve surgery turnover times, schedule cases realistically, and begin intense and proactive communication about surgery scheduling changes.

A majority of surgeon respondents (32 out of 37) said that "efficient use of their time" was very important to them. For example, surgeon's offices were often irritated with the amount of time they had to spend on the phone just to schedule a surgery slot time. At the time, the surgery center required the surgeon's office to provide a lot of patient information over the phone. The schedulers suggested changing the scheduling process so that a surgeon could reserve a spot with a few critical pieces of patient information (for example, patient's name, type of surgery). The rest of the information could be faxed later.

The survey results also helped senior managers determine appropriate capital equipment decisions. Based on the feedback received from gynecologists and

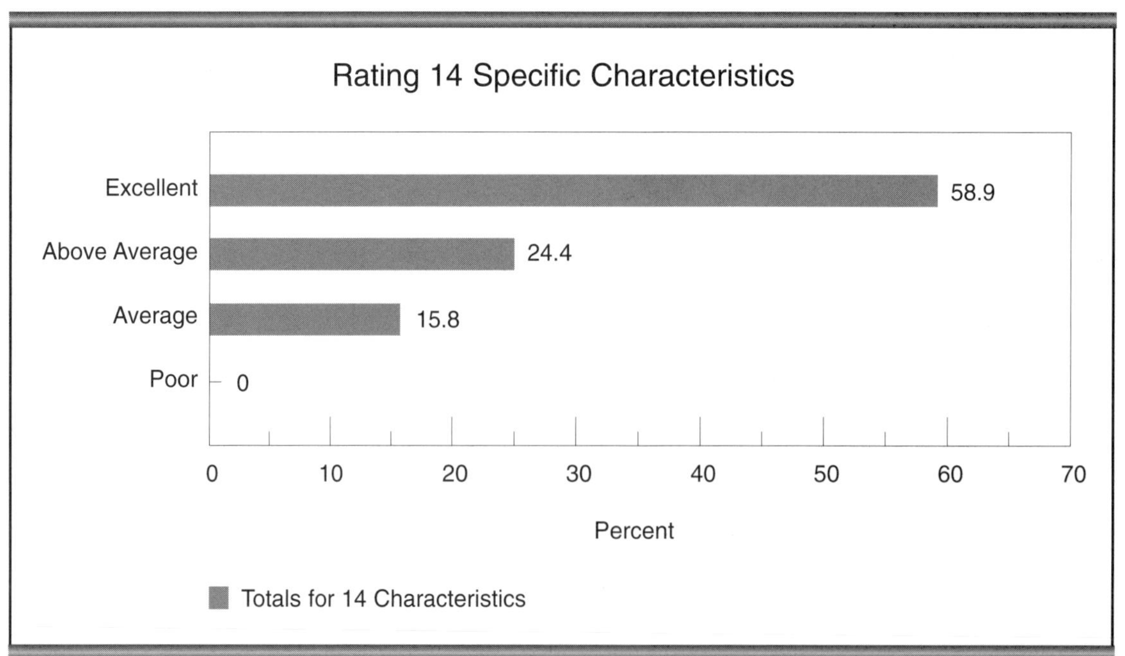

Figure 3-6. The majority of surgeons surveyed rated the surgery center as excellent or above average in 14 characteristics, including cost and responsiveness to needs. *Source:* Tallahassee Single Day Surgery Center, Tallahassee, FL. Used with permission.

plastic surgeons, equipment and instruments were evaluated and new purchases were made.

Follow-Up Survey

When surgeons were resurveyed in 1994, gynecologists rated the instruments and equipment at Tallahassee Single Day Surgery higher than other facilities. An increase in surgeon satisfaction with surgery start times was also realized. Twenty-four surgeons rated Tallahassee Single Day Surgery as excellent or above average in this area. Tallahassee Single Day Surgery plans on conducting a third physician satisfaction survey. Additional questions will be added to measure surgeons' satisfaction with how well Tallahassee communicates with medical offices and meets patients' needs and expectations.

Example 3-3. Monitoring Infection Rates at an Endoscopy Center

The Setting and Background

The Falls City Endoscopy Center is a hypothetical endoscopy center located in a New Jersey. It is an independent facility jointly owned by six gastroenterologists. Twenty other physicians from the city and surrounding areas also use the facility to perform endoscopy procedures, including colonoscopies, polypectomies, biopsies, and sigmoidoscopies.

Monitoring Infection Rates

As part of performance improvement activities, the endoscopy center continuously monitors several areas including infection rates, unplanned hospital admissions, prolonged recovery, and mortality and morbidity rates.

A nurse oversees the center's infection control program in addition to risk management and performance improvement activities. On a regular basis, she monitors device-related infections, communicable diseases such as HIV/AIDS and hepatitis, and other infections.

The endoscopy center uses a by exception method to report infections. When patients return to the endoscopy center for a follow-up visit after a procedure, staff note device-related infections and fill out a special form whenever an infection is present. These forms are then sent to the infection control nurse. Once a month, she compiles these reports and documents the number of infections to the total number of procedures performed.

Identifying and Analyzing Trends

During the last few months, the infection control nurse has noticed a small increase in the number of IV site infections. When she stratifies these data by procedure, provider, and surgical suite, she notices that 86% of the infections are occurring in patients who use Surgical Suites A and B.

The infection control nurse meets with the nurse manager to discuss the trend in IV site infections. Concerned, the nurse manager theorizes that the problem might be related to a turnover in staff. A new nurse, hired three months ago, has been primarily assigned to Suites A and B. The nurse manager questions whether this new nurse has a good understanding of infection control policies and procedures, particularly with regard to IV management.

The next day, the infection control nurse and the nurse manager observe how this new nurse inserts and removes IVs for several patients. They note that she does not follow proper procedure.

Improvement Action

The nursing manager agrees to train the new nurse in the proper procedure for handling IVs. She will then ask the new nurse to demonstrate this procedure and check her competency. The infection control nurse then sends a report of her findings to the center's performance improvement committee and informs them that the nursing manager is providing appropriate education to her staff.

The next quarter, the infection control nurse notes a decrease in the number of IV site infections. When she stratifies the data according to surgical suites, she finds that Surgical Suites A and B had no IV site infections that quarter.

Example Highlights

Setting:
Falls City Endoscopy Center, Anycity, New Jersey

Performance Improvement Initiative:
Monitor and reduce rate of nosocomial infections.

Dimensions of Performance Addressed:
Continuity, effectiveness, safety.

Comments:
This example illustrates infection control rates as one of many quality control measures that organizations monitor on an ongoing basis. Once an increasing trend is noticed in device-related infections, staff can take appropriate steps to reduce infection rates and monitor improvement.

References

The Measurement Mandate: On the Road to Performance Improvement in Health Care. Oakbrook Terrace, IL: Joint Commission on Accreditation of Healthcare Organizations, 1993.

National Library of Healthcare Indicators: Health Plan and Network Edition. Oakbrook Terrace, IL: Joint Commission on Accreditation of Healthcare Organizations, 1997.

Primer on Indicator Development and Application. Oakbrook Terrace, IL: Joint Commission on Accreditation of Healthcare Organizations, 1990.

CHAPTER 4: Assess

Chapter Highlights

Why Do We Assess?

- To compare performance with various reference points;
- To determine root causes for current performance;
- To set improvement priorities; and
- To determine the effect of improvement actions.

What Do We Assess?

- Organization performance and care outcomes;
- Initial assessment of ongoing measurement; and
- Intensive assessment triggered
- by important single events,

  –by certain performance levels and/or patterns or trends,

  –when the organization's performance varies significantly from that of other organizations,

  –when the organization's performance varies significantly from recognized standards, and

  –when the organization wishes to improve already acceptable performance.

Continued on page 88.

Continued from page 87.

Who Performs the Assessment?

- Groups that include the process owners, customers, and suppliers, with additional expert input as needed.

Assessment Techniques

- Comparing performance with important reference points, including patterns of performance, external databases, practice guidelines/parameters, and desired performance specifications or thresholds.
- Identifying best practices.

Assessment Tools

- Run charts, control charts, histograms, flowcharts, cause-and-effect diagrams, scatter diagrams, Pareto charts, selection grids, and multivoting.

Examples of Assessment

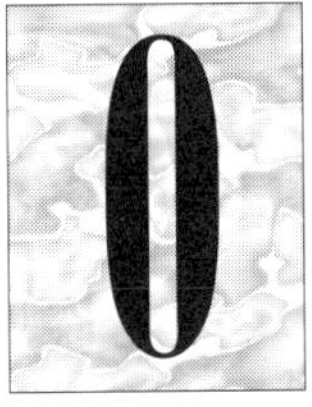

nce data are collected as part of measurement, they must be translated into information and used. Organizations can use such information to make judgments and draw conclusions about performance. This assessment forms the basis for actions taken to improve performance. Assessment activities include identifying the root causes of problems, determining the current performance, and interpreting any variations in process or outcomes that suggest that improvement may be necessary.

Figure 4-1, below, illustrates assessment's role in the improvement cycle. One vital function of assessment is the use of comparative information and internal organization data to set improvement priorities. This also may include benchmarking activities.

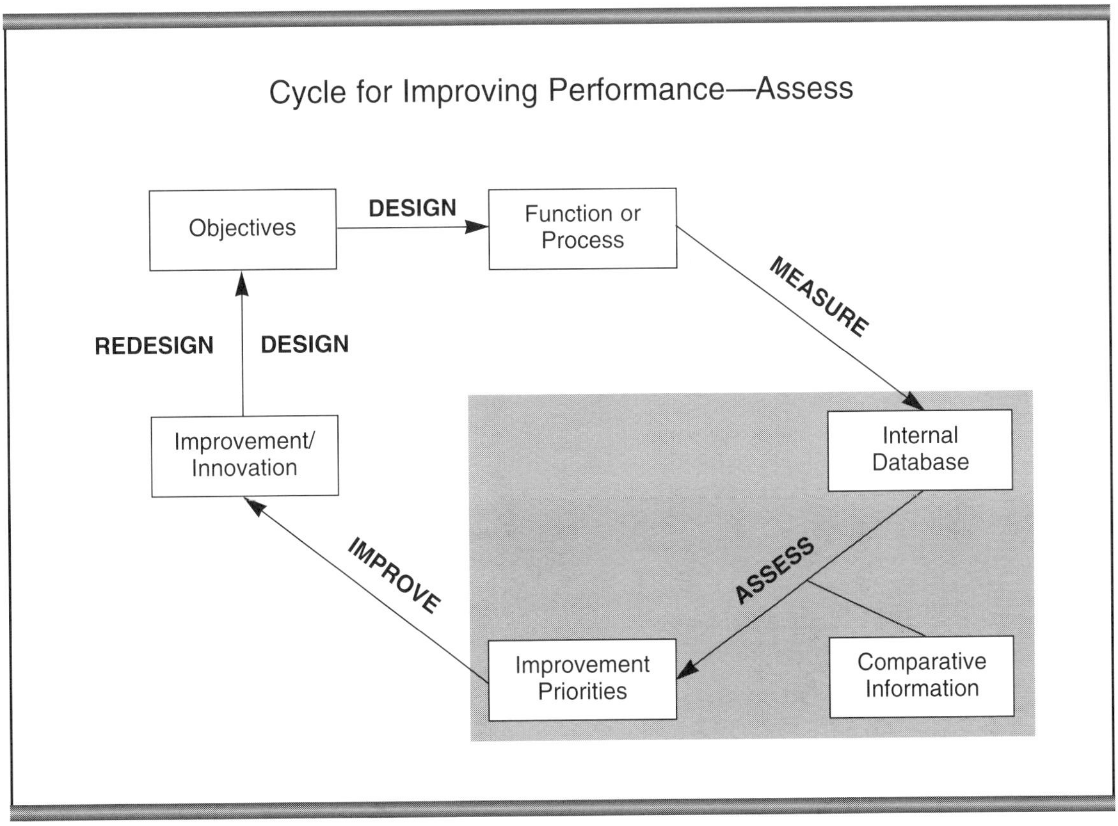

Cycle for Improving Performance—Assess

Objectives
DESIGN
Function or Process
MEASURE
Internal Database
ASSESS
Comparative Information
Improvement Priorities
IMPROVE
Improvement/ Innovation
REDESIGN
DESIGN

Figure 4-1. This figure highlights the assessment stage of the cycle for improving performance. It includes the comparative information this activity requires and the improvement priorities that result.

This chapter answers several essential questions about assessment:

- Why do we assess performance?
- What do we assess?
- Who assesses performance?
- What techniques and tools can we use to assess performance?

Why Do We Assess?

Assessment activities answer these questions:

- What are the problems that need to be solved?
- What processes or functions can we improve?
- What are the priorities among these opportunities for improvement?

Assessment is particularly important when a new process is developed. When an ambulatory care organization designs a new process, it should measure its performance and compare the resulting data to design specifications and customer expectations to determine if the process is performing well.

As a new process is designed or an existing process redesigned, it is important to include a variety of process measurement, including

- process stability;
- process capability; and
- process outcome.

After variation has been determined, assessment of data can identify the size and the types of variation and point out potential opportunities for improvement. Even if a process is stable, assessment might reveal additional possible opportunities for improvement. However, because of limited time and resources, organizations will not be able to take action to address all improvement opportunities and, therefore, must prioritize improvement opportunities.

Once an organization determines that an improvement effort is warranted, it must identify the root causes that lead to less-than-acceptable performance. These causes will be the prime targets for any improvement actions.

After an organization takes action to improve performance, it must continue to collect and assess data to determine whether improvement occurred; that is, whether undesirable variation was reduced or eliminated or whether the capability of the process and associated outcomes were improved.

An important aspect of the framework for improving performance is the recognition that performance will increasingly be viewed in the context of local, state, national, and global benchmarks. Assessment is not confined to information gathered within the walls of a single ambulatory care organization or even a collection of facilities under a larger single health care system. To better understand its level of performance, an organization or system needs to compare its performance against reference databases, professional standards, trade association guidelines, and other sources. It is also important to recognize that these standards are also dynamic and ever changing, requiring a constant comparative process.

What Do We Assess?

Assessment can be divided into two types. Routine assessment uses data from ongoing measurement, and special assessment is part of focused improvement efforts.

Routine Assessment

Data from all ongoing measurement should be assessed. How often assessment occurs depends on the process being measured, the organization's priorities, and the nature and types of indicators. For example, an imaging center may assess patient complaints immediately, whereas it may assess data pertaining to patient education every quarter. Similarly an organization might review data about child immunization rates every two months and data about staff satisfaction once a year. Routine assessment should always be reviewed from the standpoint of "How often to measure? How often to review?"

Special Assessment

At times, routine assessment will suggest that a more intensive study of a process is warranted. This could include more detailed measurement and assessment, more frequent data collection intervals, use of secondary analysis of other data relevant to the process, or more intensive analysis of the data available. More intensive assessment (or measurement and assessment) is typically triggered under the following conditions:

- By important single events, such as those identified by sentinel-event indicators (for example, a serious injury to a patient, a significant treatment complication, an unexpected hospital admission);

- By a performance level that varies significantly from an absolute level established by the organization, sometimes called a "threshold for evaluation";
- By patterns or trends that significantly vary from those expected, based on appropriate statistical analysis (for example, initiating a more intensive assessment when performance is two or more standard deviations below the mean);
- When the organization's performance significantly varies from that of other organizations or from recognized standards; and
- When the organization wishes to improve already acceptable performance levels.

The Joint Commission's standards for ambulatory care also identify some outcomes that should trigger more in-depth assessment:

- Major discrepancies, or patterns of discrepancies, between preoperative and postoperative diagnoses, including those identified during the pathologic review of specimens removed during surgical procedures;
- Confirmed transfusion reactions;
- Significant adverse drug reactions;
- Significant medication errors; and
- Significant adverse events associated with anesthesia use.

Each state may have a list of critical adverse events requiring reporting as well.

Who Performs the Assessment?

Both routine and special assessment may be performed by a number of staff and consumers. Routine assessment is typically performed by those who designed the measurement method or by others with a solid knowledge of statistics, the process being measured, the reference points against which performance is compared, or the criteria for triggering more intensive special assessment.

Special assessment ordinarily includes the people closest to the process being addressed—those who carry out or are affected by the process. Remember also the importance of cross-discipline/cross-service quality improvement efforts when considering who performs the assessment. Service, discipline, or office-location barriers cannot be allowed to limit participation in improvement efforts. When a process involves more than one service, the group improving the process should reflect all services. By including the process's participants and sometimes consumers, the ambulatory care organization not only taps the necessary expertise, it also helps ensure the necessary understanding and support for the recommended changes.

Assessment Techniques

The primary goals of assessment are to determine in what areas performance can be improved, to set priorities for improvement, and to evaluate the effectiveness of actions taken to improve performance. In general, this requires some review of the organization's performance outcome, comparisons with the performance of other organizations, and possibly identification of local or national "best practices."

Comparing Data

Most types of assessment require comparing data to some point of reference. The reference points may include:

- Historical patterns of performance in an organization and, if available, with internal longitudinal databases;
- Aggregate external reference databases;
- Practice guidelines or parameters, and clinical pathways or protocols;
- Desired performance targets, specifications, or thresholds; and
- Expected outcomes.

Historical patterns of performance in the organization. When an organization has accumulated sufficient data, it will be able to compare its current performance to its own historical patterns. This allows the organization, in effect, to act as its own control group and evaluate performance. For example, an organization might compare current performance levels with levels taken from the previous year. It could also compare performance levels for various days of the week, shifts, or parts of the organization. With good data over a significant time period, an organization can develop its own standard error of measurement estimates and empirical guidelines to help define control limits for a given process.

Perhaps one of the most common and useful comparisons using historical data involves analyzing the variation in the process. Variation is inherent in every process; performance measured by indicators will never be static. Consider, for example, that an organization is measuring turnaround time for completion of stat laboratory requests. The turnaround time cannot be identical for each laboratory test conducted, but should conform to basic expectations. In another example, consider a managed care organization that is measuring the effect of a health promotion program (such as, weight management or smoking cessation) or a social support program (such as, for depression). Obviously, not all participants will show the same result. In other words, results will vary.

Distinguishing the type of variation is important. Each type of variation will require a different type of action for improvement. Variation has two general types and causes: common-cause and special-cause. *Common-cause variation* is the random variation inherent in every process. In the smoking cessation example, each participant has a variety of personal factors that affect his or her ability to stop smoking: working conditions, family support, smoking history, and so forth. A process that varies only because of common causes is said to be *stable.* A stable process, one with only common cause variation, can be improved.

Special-cause variation arises from unusual circumstances or events that may be difficult to anticipate. This cause results in marked variation and an unstable process. Human error and mechanical malfunction are examples of special causes that result in variation. In the smoking cessation example, for instance, a special cause of variation might be a batch of faulty or ineffective nicotine patches that has been dispensed to patients. Special causes of variation must be systematically identified and eliminated. However, removing a special cause will only eliminate aberrant performance, not improve the basic level of performance. A much more fundamental improvement comes from studying the process and improving its design. Failure to distinguish the types of variation can lead to two types of errors: reacting to special-cause variation as if it were common and reacting to common-cause variation as if it were special. Both types of errors are common.

Aggregate external reference databases. In addition to assessing its own historical patterns of performance, an organization should compare its performance with that of other organizations. This kind of comparison will be increasingly important in the future when access to organization data across the country is facilitated through more advanced telecommunications. Expanding the scope of comparison helps an organization draw conclusions about its own performance and learn about different methods to design and carry out new processes.

Aggregate external databases take various forms, such as the Joint Commission's IMSystem.® Aggregate, risk-adjusted data about specific indicators produced by these databases can help each organization set priorities for improvement by showing whether its current performance falls within an expected range.

National multioffice systems often have systemwide databases that feed back information about certain indicators (for example, patient outcomes, patient satisfaction, or utilization data; the average number of visits by discipline category and patient diagnosis) to regional or branch offices for use in their individual performance improvement activities. Hospital-based ambulatory care that is part of a larger health system may initiate collection of similar data for comparison with other ambulatory organizations. Several state and federal professional or trade associations have recently initiated comparative databases in which members may participate. Typically, payers also gather information about performance and cost, as do states and the federal government.

Practice guidelines/parameters. Practice guidelines/parameters, critical paths, and other standardized client care procedures are also very useful reference points for comparison. Whether developed by professional societies, in-house practitioners, or clusters of health care organizations, these procedures represent an expert consensus about the expected practices for a given diagnosis or treatment. Examples include the recent guidelines for acute low back problems advanced by the U.S. Department of Health and Human Services Agency for Health Care Policy and Research (AHCPR). The guidelines include a guide for both clinicians and clients. Assessment variation from such established procedures can help an organization identify opportunities for improvement and build the foundation for research.

Desired performance targets. Organizations may also establish targets, specifications, or thresholds for evaluation against which they compare current performance. Such levels can be derived from professional literature or expert opinion within the organization. For example, an organization may set the following targets for patients with depression, based on the clinical literature, available depression research, and past organization performance:

- "Primary care physicians who treat depressed patients should refer those patients to a mental health professional if they do not respond to treatment within 12 weeks (AHCPR Guidelines, 1993)"; and

- "95% of all depressed patients recommended for a medication trial must receive an adequate trial of antidepressant medication as evidenced by appropriate therapeutic levels and time course."

Assessment and improvement activities would strive to help the organization create new processes or redesign existing ones to meet those targets.

Benchmarking

One method of comparing performance is benchmarking. Benchmarking is the process by which one organization studies the exemplary performance of a similar process in a similar organization and, to the greatest extent possible, adapts that information for its own use. Although a benchmark can be any point of comparison, most often it is a standard of excellence. Xerox, a winner of the Malcolm Baldrige National Quality Award in 1989, defines benchmarking as "the search for the industry's best practices that lead to superior performance." An organization may also look to nonhealth care organizations to identify best practices, including hotels, automotive manufacturers, and so forth.

Organizations can also use an informal version of benchmarking, sometimes called comparative data analysis, to compare their results with those of other organizations or with current research or literature. For example, a primary care clinic wanting to study its processes for employee recognition and retention might want to review local, state, or national trends on employee attrition in the work force. Or an endoscopy center may want to compare the adequacy of its colon preparation rates to those of other providers.

Studying the patterns of care or service in another organization often results in an infusion of new ideas—ideas that never would have arisen if the assessment and comparison remained within one's own walls. The organization serving as the benchmark or "best practice" model can benefit as well. By discussing the process in question—by reexamining each step and its rationale—the organization may also gain new insights. Figure 4-2, page 97, illustrates one approach to successful benchmarking.

Assessing Factors That Affect Performance

More intensive assessment requires learning what factors cause the current performance and its relationship to the outcomes. This is achieved by studying a process; learning its steps and critical decision points; identifying the various people, actions, and equipment required for the process's outcomes; finding

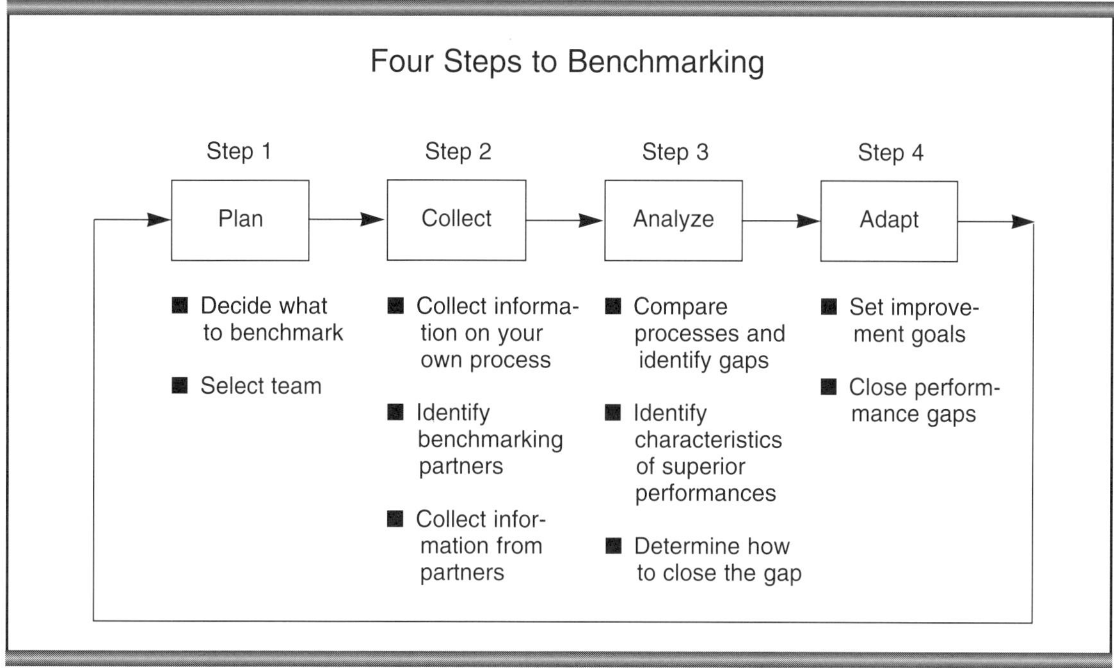

Figure 4-2. This figure illustrates one approach to benchmarking.
Source: **Flower J: Benchmarking. Springboard or buzzword? *Healthc Forum* 36(1):14–16, 1993. Reprinted with permission.**

links among variables in performance; and ranking the frequency of causes. Tools such as flowcharts, cause-and-effect diagrams, and Pareto charts described later in this chapter are useful in studying a process and identifying potential areas for improvement.

Setting Priorities for Improvement

Setting priorities for measurement and improvement is a critical step in any quality effort. Throughout the improvement cycle, organization leaders must set priorities for deciding what to measure, what to assess, and what to improve. Deciding what to improve is perhaps most important because of the significant investment of time and effort involved as well as the potential effect on organizationwide performance.

An ambulatory care organization's leaders play a key role in setting priorities for improvement. Leaders are in the best position to view the organization's overall goals, the availability of resources to address the improvement opportunities, and the organizationwide effect of change in process and outcome. Priority-setting decisions should reflect ambulatory care research, expert judgment, and information. They combine epidemiology, diagnostic understanding, therapeutic efficacy, and anticipated cost/benefit of improvement. Leaders, of course, need input from the appropriate people and departments, units, teams, and offices in the organization.

Priorities for improvement are dynamic and ever changing. They can be influenced in various ways, such as

- a sentinel event that requires immediate improvement action;
- a new or modified strategic direction from the governing body or organization leadership;
- the initiation of a new service or service location;
- a change in the organization's structure, such as by a joint venture or acquisition;
- client/family feedback;
- recent clinical developments and innovations;
- referral source, physician, staff, community, or payer feedback; and
- legislative and community health care reform actions.

An organized approach to setting the priorities for improvement should be as objective and comprehensive as possible. Organizations might consider creating a set of selection criteria to use in this process that indicate a range of organization priorities. The following list suggests possible selection criteria:

- ***The degree to which the opportunity reflects the organization's mission, philosophy, goals, and policies.*** If, for example, one of a surgical center's key strategic goals is to increase the number of surgical cases performed, then leaders might focus on improving areas of performance that are important to local surgeons and would make them want to use the center (for example, simplified administrative processes).
- ***Whether the resources required to pursue the improvement opportunity are available.*** Some improvements, such as minor procedural changes, require relatively few resources; others require more substantial amounts of time (for example, creating a critical path, redesigning a clinical service) and funds (for example, establishing a new service, opening a new branch location). The resources required must be weighed against the resources available and the benefits expected. In some cases, the lack of resources necessary to make an improvement will result in the opportunity being assigned a lower priority.

- ***Whether the opportunity affects one of the patient care and organization functions identified in the Joint Commission's standards.*** These functions include assessment of patients, education of patients and families, and management of the environment of care. How well these functions are carried out significantly affects the care clients receive and the organization's ability to provide that care.
- ***Whether the improvement opportunity addresses a high-volume, high-risk, or problem-prone process.*** For example, a high-volume process for many ambulatory care organizations is likely to be clinical assessment and education efforts. A high-risk process might be administering anesthesia. A problem-prone activity might be patient waiting times.
- ***The degree to which the opportunity reflects patients' priorities with respect to their needs, preferences, and expectations.*** In an ambulatory care organization, patients and their care givers are critical customers. It is essential to know what their needs and health care experiences have been.
- ***Whether the opportunity pertains to a high-impact clinical service.*** An endoscopy center might identify colonoscopy as a high-impact service, whereas a pediatric clinic might identify immunizations as a high impact service.
- ***Whether the opportunity pertains to utilization management, risk management, and/or quality control concerns.*** These areas are typically of high priority in a health care organization. For example, a quality control concern might be adverse drug reactions in an oncology center or the accuracy of IV mixture in a surgery center.
- ***Whether the opportunity addresses a high-cost function or process, or whether the opportunity promises significant cost savings.*** The pressing need to provide care efficiently makes potentially cost-saving changes high-priority opportunities. An example for any ambulatory care organization would be training and retraining qualified staff. By improving its processes for staff orientation and ongoing training, the organization might find that it is able to retain its experienced staff, thus saving the costs of frequently recruiting and orienting new staff. It might also improve staff ability to function in key areas (for example, life safety, patient care functions).
- ***Whether the opportunity for improvement represents a cross-discipline, cross-functional aspect of performance.*** The evolving Joint Commission standards and experience in quality improvement efforts emphasize the importance of cross-discipline, cross-functional care delivery.

Selection grids and multivoting are useful tools for setting priorities and making team decisions. They are discussed later in this chapter.

Assessing Individual Performance

Most widespread and fundamental improvement arises from attention to processes and systems. However, at times, measurement and assessment will also identify individual performance as the cause of variation. In that case, intensive assessment, review and recommendation, and any appropriate action and follow up are required.

Each organization is expected to have detailed procedures for addressing a problem in an individual's performance (for example, individual counseling, education, responsibility changes, required consultation). The organization's leaders are also responsible for assessing the competence of staff members.

Although individual performance issues will continue to arise, it is vital to remember these tenets of performance improvement:

- Ambulatory care professionals are skilled, knowledgeable, and dedicated;
- The vast majority of improvement opportunities lie in processes, not individuals; and
- Some of the best opportunities for improvement lie in integrative work (for example, connections between different services for the same patient over time) and core processes.

Assessment Tools

For continuous improvement of health care, tools and methods are needed that document observations, build knowledge, and share understanding with others. This section provides a quick overview of a few tools and methods for performance assessment within the scientific approach. These simple but powerful tools can be learned quickly and utilized effectively by all organization members.

Statistical Tools

Three statistical quality control tools are especially helpful in comparing performance with historical patterns and assessing variation and stability: run charts, control charts, and histograms.

Run charts. A run chart (also known as a time plot) plots points on a graph to illustrate levels of performance over time. It also demonstrates a trend, such as movement away from the average. It can help identify which existing processes need improvement and can show whether an action taken to improve performance was successful. Figure 4-3, below, plots the average turnaround time for Pap smears for each month in 1996. Leaders with system knowledge can use run charts to track operating indicators.

Control charts. Adding computed limits (control limits) to a chart increases the value of a longitudinal record. A control chart is a run chart with the addi-

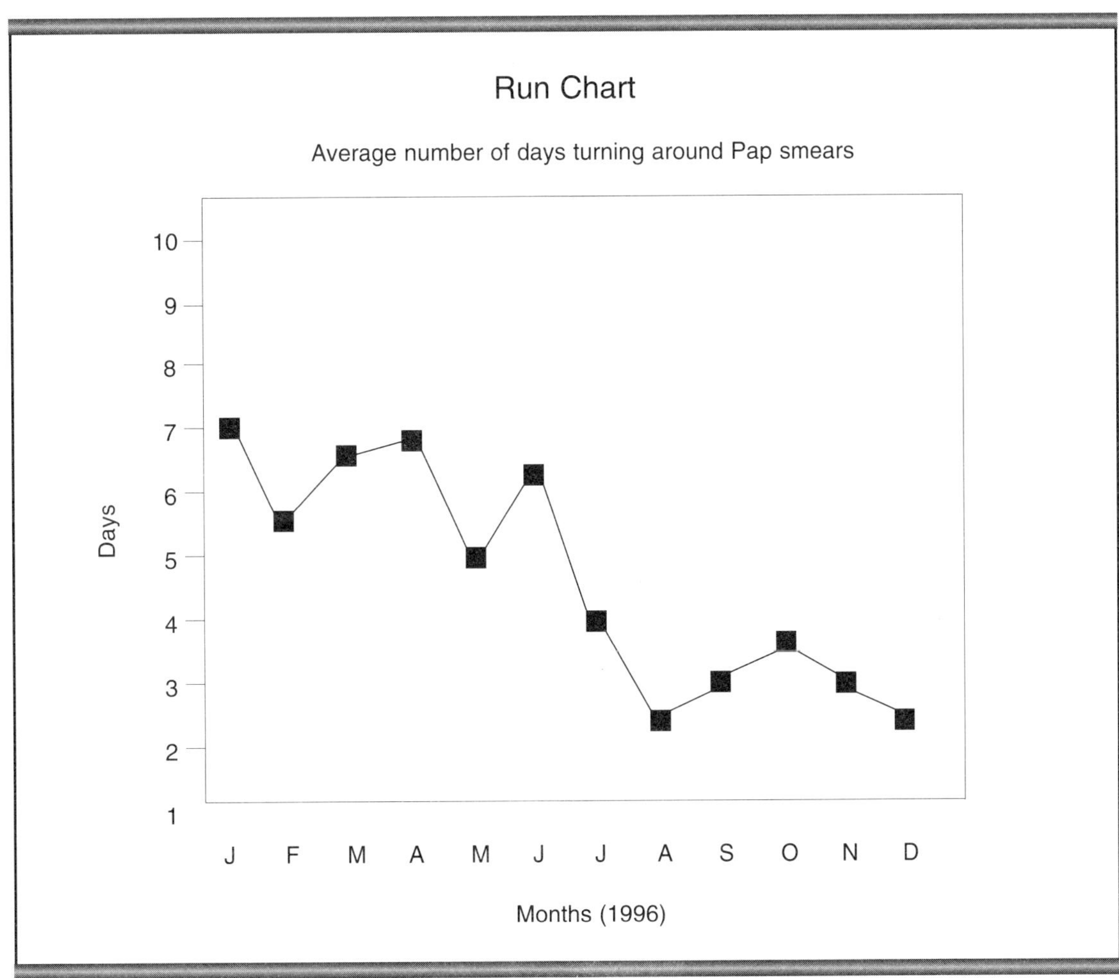

Figure 4-3. A run chart displays points on a graph to show levels of performance over time.

tion of a statistically derived upper control limit (UCL) and lower control limit (LCL). It shows variation in a process and helps discern whether that variation is due to special or common causes. When performance variation is random and stays within the UCL and LCL, the causes of the variation are considered common causes. When performance exceeds the upper or lower control limits, or demonstrates specific predictable patterns within the control limits, the variation is due to a special cause. Figure 4-4, below, shows an example of a control chart. It is important to note that control limits are not the same as specification limits, budgets, targets, goals, or objectives. They only indicate what the process is capable of, not what the process is expected to perform or what the process designers hope to achieve.

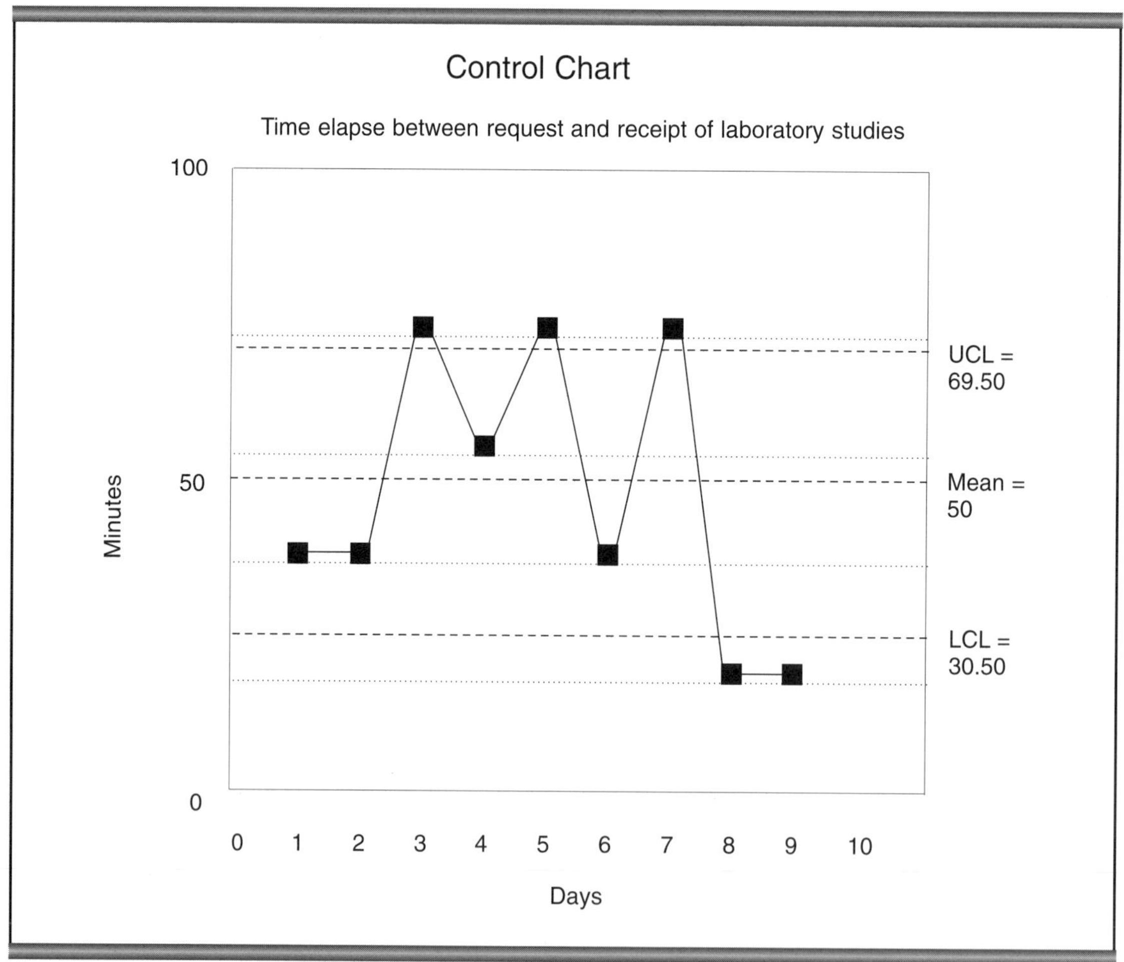

Figure 4-4. A control chart indicates if a process is statistically in control.

Histograms. Histograms show the pattern of variation in a process or its outcomes. For example, patient waiting time can range from four to fifty minutes. This variation may seem unpredictable, but it generally follows some pattern; the range of variation is predictable. In most cases, the variation is expected to fall within a normal distribution. For example, perhaps waiting time (for non-emergencies) is expected to be 15 minutes. At times, however, the waiting time is not normal and is unpredictable. This may signal the need for further evaluation. Histograms illustrate these ranges of variation. Figure 4-5, below, gives an example of a histogram along with instructions on creating one. The histogram is also related to the Pareto chart discussed on page 107.

Causal and Process Analysis

A number of tools are helpful for determining the root causes of current performance: flowcharts, cause-and-effect diagrams, scatter diagrams, and Pareto charts.

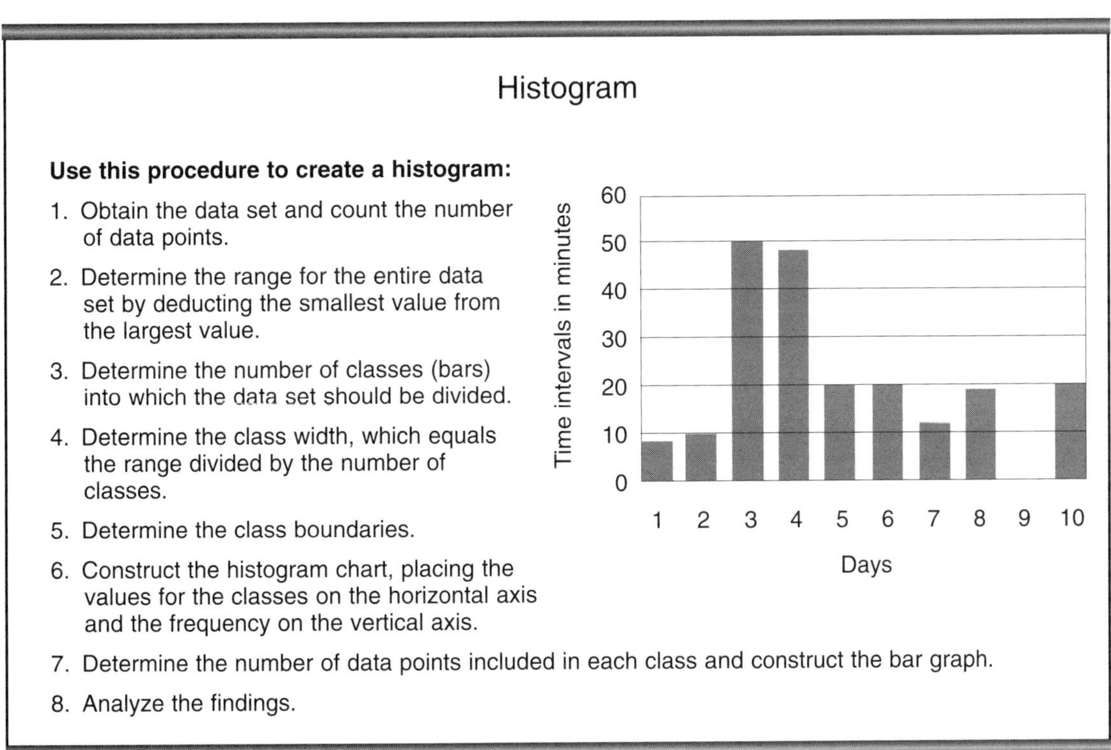

Figure 4-5. A histogram helps organizations discover patterns of variation in processes and outcomes.

Flowcharts. Flowcharts are visual schematics that show step-by-step the unfolding of a process or a plan of an activity. A flowchart identifies the actual path that a process follows, as opposed to the one that may be defined in the policies and procedures manual. Flowcharts may include top-down flowcharts, detailed flowcharts, workflow diagrams, and deployment charts. By documenting a process's sequence in steps in a flowchart, a team can identify redundancies, inefficiencies, misunderstandings, endless loops, waiting times, and inspection steps that are the areas that create the biggest problems in most processes. This helps the team gain an understanding about how the process should be performed. Once the actual process is illustrated in the flowchart, the team can create a flowchart to show the ideal path the process should take. In many organizations processes are being used that have never been described or fully studied, but have grown out of historical practice patterns.

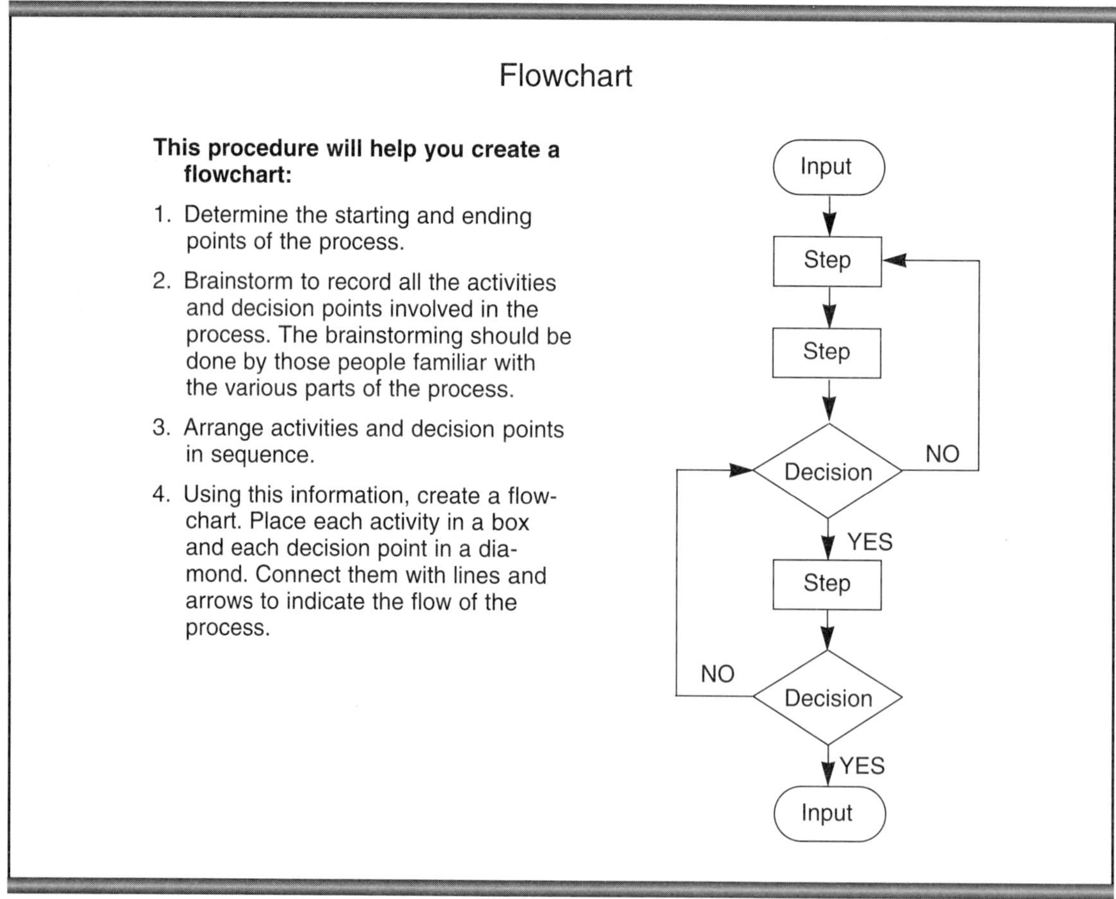

Figure 4-6. A flowchart illustrates the sequence of steps that a process follows.

Teams can use flowcharts at several crucial stages, such as

- designing new processes;
- designing a method for measuring a process;
- identifying problems;
- analyzing problems to determine causes; and
- planning solutions.

See Figure 4-6, page 104, for an example of how to create a flowchart.

Cause-and-effect diagrams. A cause-and-effect diagram is sometimes called a "fishbone" diagram (because of its shape) or an Ishikawa diagram (after its creator, Kaoru Ishikawa). It enables the team to map out a list of factors thought to affect a problem or desired outcome. It can show a large number of possible causes of a particular outcome (sometimes negative outcomes, such as delays, medication errors, client dissatisfaction). It is constructed using the experience and expertise of the process's customers and suppliers, and it shows how various components of the process relate to one another. Once completed, the diagram helps identify specific conditions requiring further attention and might suggest appropriate actions. A cause-and-effect diagram can provide ideas for

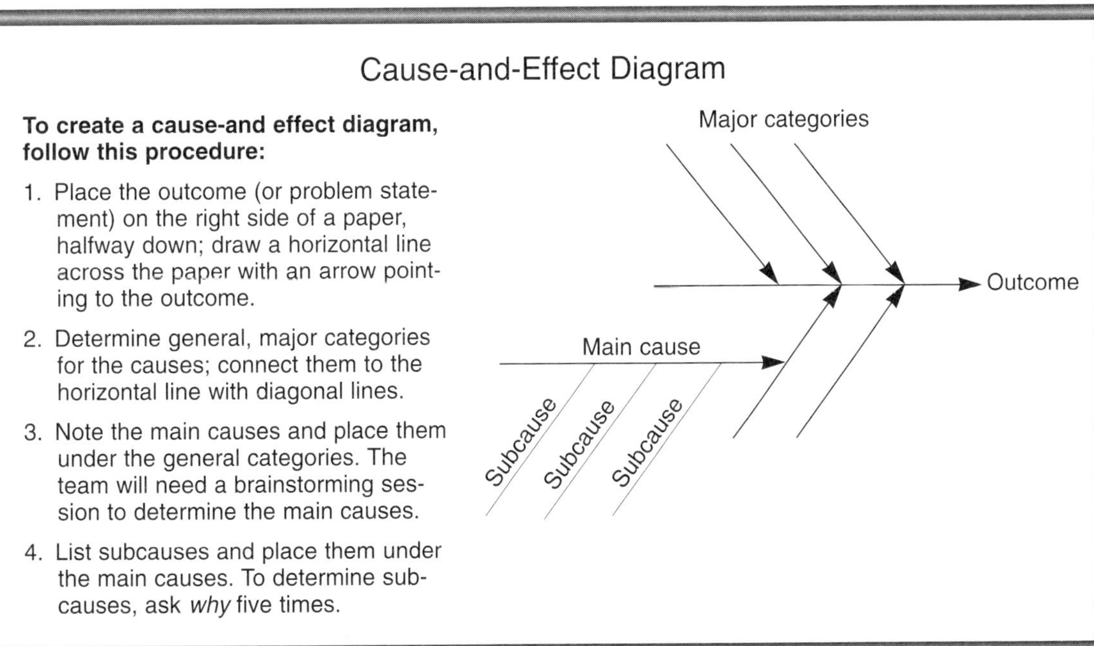

To create a cause-and effect diagram, follow this procedure:

1. Place the outcome (or problem statement) on the right side of a paper, halfway down; draw a horizontal line across the paper with an arrow pointing to the outcome.
2. Determine general, major categories for the causes; connect them to the horizontal line with diagonal lines.
3. Note the main causes and place them under the general categories. The team will need a brainstorming session to determine the main causes.
4. List subcauses and place them under the main causes. To determine subcauses, ask *why* five times.

Figure 4-7. A cause-and-effect diagram depicts the large number of possible causes of a particular outcome.

data collection to measure performance. An example of a cause-and-effect diagram and the procedure for creating such a diagram are provided in Figure 4-7, page 105.

Scatter diagrams. Another useful assessment tool is the scatter diagram, which illustrates the statistical relationship between two variables. Groups use scatter diagrams when they want to examine a theory about the relationship between two variables, when they analyze raw data, and when they assess an action taken to improve performance.

In a scatter diagram, each variable is assigned an axis; points where the variables intersect are marked with dots. The shape of the scatter of points tells you if there is a relationship. If the points cluster in an area running from lower left to upper right, the variables have a positive correlation; if they cluster from upper left to lower right, they have a negative correlation. If there is no relationship, the points are scattered randomly over the graph. A scatter diagram may not conclusively prove a relationship, but it can offer some convincing evidence. Figure 4-8, below, gives more information on how these diagrams are created and includes a sample illustration.

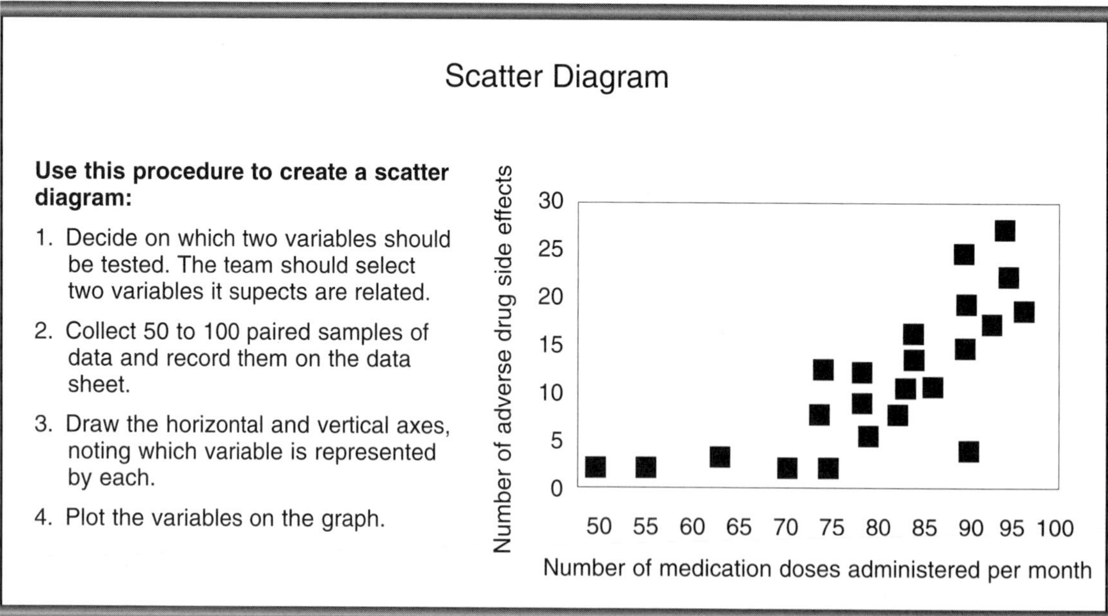

Figure 4-8. A scatter diagram illustrates the relationship between two variables.

Pareto charts. A Pareto chart depicts, in descending order, the frequency of problems affecting the process being studied. This useful bar graph allows a group to categorize occurrences and focus on those that most frequently occur and are, therefore, most important. It is a natural follow-up to a cause-and-effect diagram. Having listed a number of causes, the group could use a Pareto chart to display their relative frequency. This information would, in turn, help a group decide which cause to address first. Figure 4-9, below, displays a simple procedure for how to create a Pareto chart.

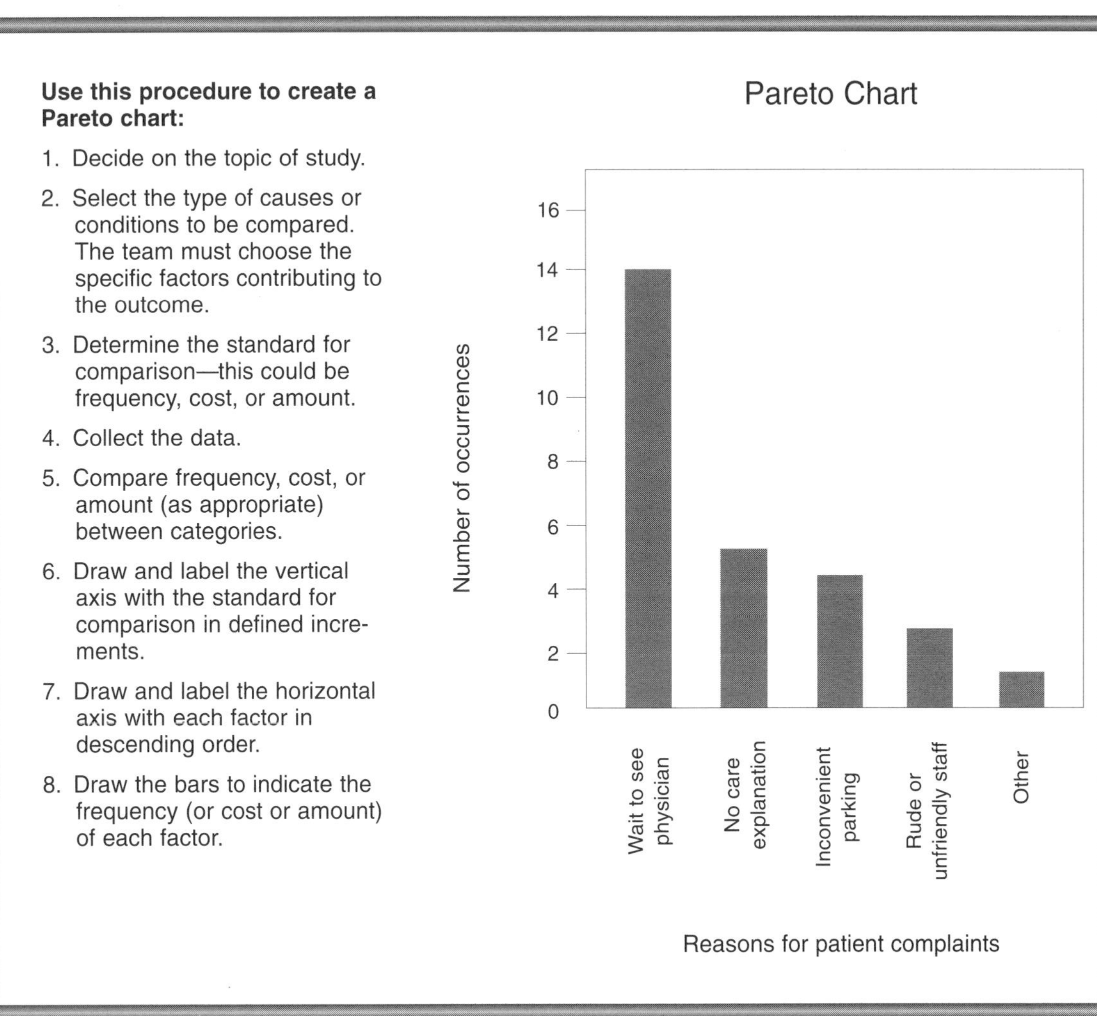

Figure 4-9. A Pareto chart depicts in descending order (from left to right) the frequency of events being studied.

Decision Making and Planning

Two specific tools can be used to set priorities for improvement and help team decision making: selection grids and multivoting.

Selection grids. A selection grid can be a useful tool for setting priorities for improvement. Figure 4-10, below, shows how this tool works. The horizontal axis of the matrix lists the selection criteria; the vertical axis lists the improvement opportunities. Each person assigns a score to indicate the effect of a particular criterion on an opportunity. The points are totaled for each opportunity;

Selection Grid

Criteria / Issues	Quality of care	Patient satisfaction	Staff morale	Cost	Total
Issue #1	X	X	—		x – 2 0 – 0 - – 1
Issue #2	0	X	X	—	x – 2 0 – 1 - – 1
Issue #3	—	X	0	X	x – 2 0 – 1 - – 1
Issue #4	—	—	X	0	x – 1 0 – 1 - – 2
Issue #5	0	—		—	x – 0 0 – 1 x – 0
Issue #6	0	0	—	X	x – 1 0 – 2 - – 1

Key to scoring:
x = strong effect 0 = some effect
— = weak effect blank = no effect

Figure 4-10. A selection grid helps set priorities for quality improvement. Each issue is examined for four criteria, with scores assigned for each. The answers can help a team see where its priorities actually lie.

higher totals suggest higher priorities. Responses to specific criteria may also help determine improvement priorities. For example, although the total was highest for issue #1, it may not be chosen as a focus for improvement if the group did not tend to agree that the issue affected the quality of patient care.

Multivoting. Another tool for setting improvement opportunities is multivoting—a technique for narrowing a broad list of ideas to those that are most important. Each person involved in the multivote has a limited number of points to assign to a predetermined list of improvement opportunities. These can be given in any number to any of the possibilities, with the num-ber indicating level of importance. Once the votes are tallied, the range of possibilities is usually narrowed to those the group considers most important. See Figure 4-11, below, for a simple procedure on how to conduct multivoting.

Multivoting

Use this procedure for multivoting:

1. Using a predetermined list of ideas, consider whether any are duplicates or similar.
2. Ask the group—especially those who identified the items in question—whether similar items may be grouped together.
3. If the group agrees, combine the duplicate or similar items.
4. Number each item on the new list.
5. Determine the number of points that will be assigned to each group member.
6. Allow several minutes for group members to independently assign their points to one or more of the items on the list.
7. Indicate each member's point allocation on the list.
8. Tally the votes for each item on the list.
9. Note the items that received the greatest number of points.
10. Choose the final group or multivote again.

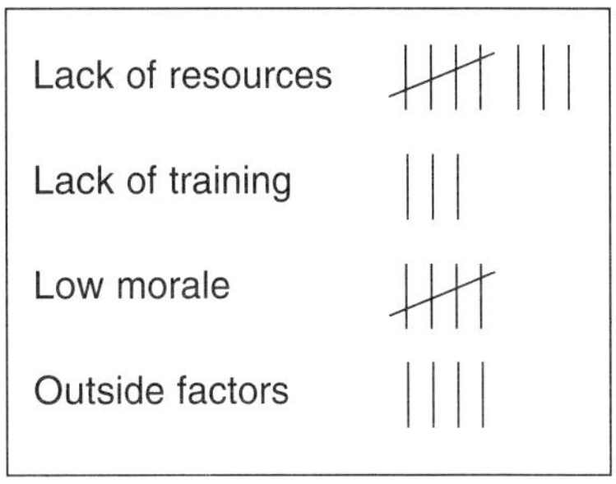

Lack of resources	~~IIII~~ III
Lack of training	III
Low morale	~~IIII~~
Outside factors	IIII

Figure 4-11. Multivoting narrows a broad list of ideas to those that are most important.

Examples of Assessment

The following examples illustrate a range of assessment projects in various ambulatory health care organizations.

Example 4-1. Assessing the Causes of Macrosomic Deliveries at a Women's Health Center

The Setting and Background

Henderson Walton Women's Center (HWWC) in Birmingham, Alabama, provides obstetrics, gynecology, and general medical services to women who live in and around Birmingham, Alabama. The center is managed by Medisphere Management Inc (MMI), a physician management organization. There are 14 physicians on staff, and in 1994, the annual patient population was 80,434.

HWWC is actively involved in performance improvement activities. Each department/service measures important aspects of care on a regular basis to ensure that they are performing as well as they think they are. Whenever a department finds that it is not performing well in a certain area, the department identifies and implements improvement actions, and measures again to see if the area has improved.

The Problem

HWWC screens pregnant women to see if they are gestationally diabetic. As reported in literature, gestational diabetics are at higher risk of having a macro-

Example Highlights

Setting:
Henderson Walton Women's Center (HWWC), Birmingham, Alabama

Performance Improvement Initiative:
Identify contributing factors of macrosomic deliveries and develop a plan to reduce the number of such deliveries.

Dimensions of Performance Addressed:
Appropriateness, availability, continuity, effectiveness, efficacy, efficiency, safety.

Comments:
This example illustrates the process of looking at a trend, identifying root causes, and planning an improvement activity.

somic baby (that is, greater than 9 lbs). Because large babies are difficult to deliver, the mother runs a higher chance of Cesarean section. Other risks include a potential trauma to the mother (tearing and lacerations) and baby (increased chance of shoulder dystocia) during delivery. There is also a small increased risk of fetal demise.

To prevent these outcomes, HWWC follows the screening procedure recommended by the American College of Obstetrics and Gynecology and the American Diabetes Association. Between the 24th and 28th week of gestation, women are given a one-hour glucose tolerance screen. If a woman's blood glucose level is greater than 140 mg/dl, she is given a second, three-hour glucose test.

A diagnosis of gestational diabetes is made when two or more venous plasma glucose concentrations are met or exceed
the following:

- fasting, 105 mg/dl;
- 1-hour, 190 mg/dl;
- 2-hour, 165 mg/dl; or
- 3-hour, 145 mg/dl.

Sandra Vinson, RD, LD, HWWC's nutritionist, gives appropriate diet instruction for a calculated diet with calories based on caloric need per kilogram of body weight. Insulin is added by physician order based on the results of the three-hour glucose tolerance test.

Despite the consistent use of these glucose screen tests, the physicians noted they were seeing a fairly large number of macrosomic deliveries. The physicians brought this to the attention of the Quality Improvement Committee.

Elesia Guyton, the obstetrics coordinator, receives delivery data from the hospital when any of the organization's patients deliver. She enters this information into the obstetrics medical record. These data are then compiled into statistics for the practice and are reviewed by the medical executive committee.

Sandra instructs patients with elevated glucose screens on how to change their diet so as to improve glucose control. She asks the obstetrics coordinator to allow her to review the delivery outcomes on all patients she has instructed and on any patient who delivers a macrosomic infant, regardless of her glucose screen results. This process allows her to review patients outcomes and assess whether providing glucose screenings and diet instruction positively affected the birth weight outcomes of infants.

While reviewing the records of patients who deliver macrosomic infants, Sandra notes a common trait: body mass index and prenatal weight gains affect infant delivery weights. She then decides to monitor delivery outcomes for one year to validate these data.

Measuring the Problem

Sandra identifies several questions: Which women are having macrosomic deliveries? Are these the women passing the glucose screen and still having large babies? Were these women identified as diabetic and provided nutrition counseling and insulin, as indicated, but still result in macrosomic deliveries?

Sandra believes that the amount of weight a woman gains during pregnancy is a contributing factor in macrosomic deliveries. This theory is supported by the literature, which states that prenatal weight gain that exceeds the recommended range of the appropriate weight category, increases the risk of management. Sandra then decides to monitor all women at HWWC who have a macrosomic delivery for the course of one year (January through December). She collects data on three groups of obstetrics patients:

- Group I. Women who have a macrosomic delivery, regardless of whether or not their 3-hour glucose test indicates they are gestationally diabetic. (These patients do no enter the study through the diet instruction process.)
- Group II. All women who have an elevated 1-hour glucose screen (using a cutoff of 140 mg/dl after 50 grams oral glucose load), but have normal results on the three-hour glucose test.
- Group III. Women who are found to be gestationally diabetic after a three-hour glucose screen and are on insulin.

To assess whether a woman's weight gain was excessive during pregnancy, Sandra uses the National Academy of Sciences' Body Mass Index (BMI) Reference as a guideline:

- Underweight women should gain 28 to 40 pounds;
- Overweight women should gain about 15 to 25 pounds; and
- Women of normal weight should gain between 25 and 30 pounds.

Findings

During 1995, a total of 105 women had macrosomic delivery outcomes (out of 1,773 deliveries). This came to 6% of the total deliveries at HWWC that year. Of those deliveries, almost all had passed the glucose screen (that is, results less than 140 mg/dl) at 24 to 28 weeks gestation. Only 11% failed the glucose test and 5% had gestational diabetes (see Figure 4-12, below).

See page 107 for a discussion on pareto charts.

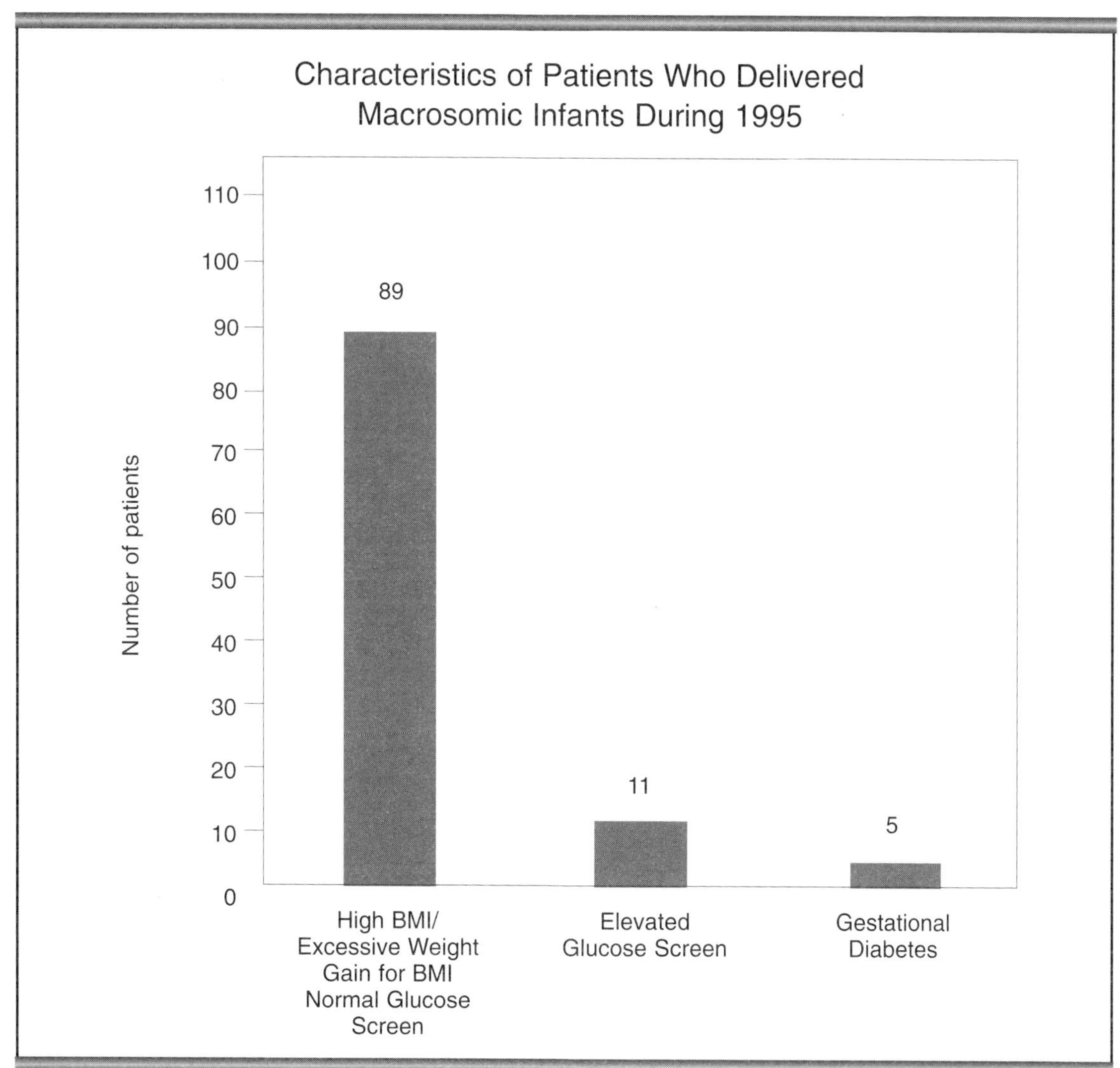

Figure 4-12. Data confirmed that excessive weight was a significant risk factor for macrosomia.
Source: **Henderson and Walton Women's Center, Birmingham, AL. Used with permission.**

When Sandra divided the women by various characteristics, she found that:

- 89 of the total 105 patients who delivered macrosomic infants had one or both risk factors of high BMI and excessive prenatal weight gain for BMI ranking;
- 33 patients (or 33%) had a family history of diabetes;
- 26 patients (or 26%) reflected an obstetrical history of macrosomia; and
- 33 patients (or 33%) had passed the glucose screen with a result of less than 140 mg/dl yet fell into the range of 120-140 mg/dl.

These data confirmed her theory that weight gain was a major risk factor for macrosomic deliveries. In fact, Sandra found that the largest distinguishing factor among macrosomic deliveries was excessive weight gain.

Weight gain was also a risk factor in women who had elevated glucose screens and were gestationally diabetic (that is, Group II and III of the study):

- In women with elevated glucose screens, 11 (11%) had macrosomic infants. Six of these women (55%) experienced excessive prenatal weight gains.
- In women who were gestationally diabetic, five (5%) had macrosomic deliveries. Three of these patients gained 17 pounds during the last 10 weeks of gestation. The other two refused their insulin.

In addition, 13 of the 14 women in both groups had glycosuria during the three-hour glucose screen (that is, they showed glucose levels above the normal range in their urine).

Assessing the Findings

After assessing the findings, Sandra drew the following conclusions:

- Pregravid weight status based on BMI, pattern of weight gain, and total weight gain emerged as factors for an increased risk for macrosomia in all groups studied;
- Patients with 1-hour glucose screen results of 120 to 140 and high BMI warrant further monitoring;
- Patients with high BMI are at a greater risk for macrosomia regardless of glucose testing results;

- Patient risk factors for macrosomia should be given special attention and guidance from those who provide care, including the physician and dietitian, regarding the nutritional support of these pregnancies and recommended weight gain patterns; and
- Glycosuria noted on obstetric 3-hour glucose screen results may warrant more attention, follow up, and guidance from the health care team.

Next Steps

Sandra will present the data to the medical executive committee and will suggest several steps to decrease macrosomia:

- A risk factor checklist and the BMI weight gain graphs could be included in the obstetrics medical record;
- When patients demonstrate a 120- to 140-mg/dl range on the 1-hour glucose screen (rather than 140 mg/dl or higher), the physician should consider giving the patient a 3-hour screen or repeating the 1-hour test based on other risk factors;
- Physicians should give special attention to weight gain during the last trimester for insulin-dependent, gestationally diabetic patients; and
- Physicians should give attention to glycosuria during the three-hour glucose screen.

Once Sandra receives physician feedback, a team will work on implementing appropriate solutions and then measure outcomes to see if the steps implemented lower the clinic's rate of macrosomia.

Example 4-2. Studying Documentation of Patient Assessment for Ambulatory Care

The Setting and Background

Hoag Memorial Hospital Presbyterian is a 416-bed hospital in Newport Beach, California. The hospital handles a high volume of outpatient procedures, including endoscopies, heart catheterizations, angiograms, and bronchoscopies. Patients are admitted to the Ambulatory Care Recovery Unit, and then are assessed, medicated, and prepared for their procedure. The patient is then transported to the appropriate treatment area. After the procedure is completed, the patient is transported back to the Ambulatory Care Recovery Unit for recovery and discharge.

Find a Process to Improve

In 1994, hospital leaders assigned task forces to assess the hospital's compli-ance with each of the Joint Commission's key functions. The organization's leaders wanted to identify areas in which the hospital could improve performance and better comply with Joint Commission requirements.

Members of the Continuum of Care Task Force determined that the current process for assessing outpatients was replete with duplicative steps, which caused unnecessary delays. Patients were often assessed twice—once in the Ambulatory Care Recovery Unit and again in the procedure area. As a result, patients were being asked the same questions several times.

The task force felt that improving the outpatient assessment process would benefit a variety of customers:

- Patients would avoid duplication of questions;
- Health care workers would avoid duplicating efforts and would be better able to communicate valid information regarding the patient;
- Physicians would benefit from fewer delays due to duplicate paperwork and from readily comparative data on the patient's condition throughout the procedure;
- Payers would have a concise record of a patient's admission; and
- Institution could save up to $20,000 in reduced printing costs, in addition to staff time and labor savings.

Example Highlights

Setting:
Hoag Memorial Hospital Presbyterian, Ambulatory Care Recovery Unit, Newport Beach, California

Performance Improvement Initiative:
Streamline the patient assessment process.

Dimensions of Performance Addressed:
Appropriateness, continuity, effectiveness, efficacy, efficiency, safety, timeliness.

Comments:
This example illustrates how a cross-departmental team uses the FOCUS-PDCA method to produce an efficient and effective patient assessment process.

Organize a Team That Knows the Process

The team was led by Mary Wong, a charge nurse from radiology, and was facilitated by Judy Bethe, the program manager for quality improvement. Other members included: the supervisor from pulmonary, the charge nurse from ambulatory care recovery, the nurse manager from the gastrointestinal laboratory, and a registered nurse from the cardiac catheter laboratory. The risk manager and the director of medical records also participated on an as-needed basis.

Clarify the Process

To better understand how outpatients were assessed at Hoag, team members made a flowchart of the process. By discussing the process, the team found that nurses in the Ambulatory Recovery Unit were using one form to assess the patient, and nurses in various procedure areas were using other forms.

See page 104 for a discussion on flowcharts.

The team then collected the patient assessment forms being used to collect and record data in the five clinical areas—pulmonary, cardiology, gastrointestinal laboratory, radiology, and the ambulatory care recovery unit.

Understand Variation

The team studied all the patient assessment forms and learned that 80% of the questions were duplicative. The team checked the forms against Joint Commission standards and found that not all the forms complied with patient assessment requirements.

To further assess the process, team members developed and distributed a staff satisfaction survey and found that the procedure staff were not satisfied with the current process because they realized that much of the information they were collecting was redundant and the process was time consuming.

The team also assessed patient satisfaction with the current process. Team members reviewed outpatient satisfaction questionnaires for comments relating to redundancy of questions. They discovered that it made some patients nervous to be asked three times whether they are allergic to any medications.

To assess the efficiency of the current system, the team calculated how long it took nurses, on average, to gather and document patient assessment information over a one-week period. The average time varied in the five clinical areas, from a low of 6.7 minutes in the gastrointestinal laboratory to a high of 18.4 minutes for the initial assessment in the ambulatory care recovery unit (see Figure 4-13, page 119). In some cases, the team found that nurses were unable to complete documentation by the conclusion of the patient's procedure.

See page 103 for a discussion on histograms.

Select and Plan the Improvement

After reviewing the data, the team agreed that it was feasible to create one patient assessment and procedure form that all five clinical areas would use (see Figure 4-14, pages 120–121). The team decided that the form should have two sections: one that includes all the common questions being asked, and a second section that has specific questions for various procedures (for example, pulmonary, angiography, cardiology).

The registered nurses in the ambulatory care recovery unit initiated the form and sent it with the patient to the procedure area via the patient record. The next nurse verified the information by initialing the previous assessment.

The team designed the form to reduce documentation time. The form used check boxes to record expected outcomes and was designed so nurses can easily record normal patient progress and still have room to document the unexpected or unusual.

Improvement Review

Team members circulated the draft form to their respective departments. Since each department was represented on the team, this helped the various departments accept the changes proposed by the team. The hospital's Forms Committee also reviewed the form and identified configuration issues to ensure that it was cost efficient to produce and met the requirements of the medical records department. The new form replaced 11 individual forms and resulted in a $20,000 reduction in printing costs, in addition to reduced staff time and labor costs.

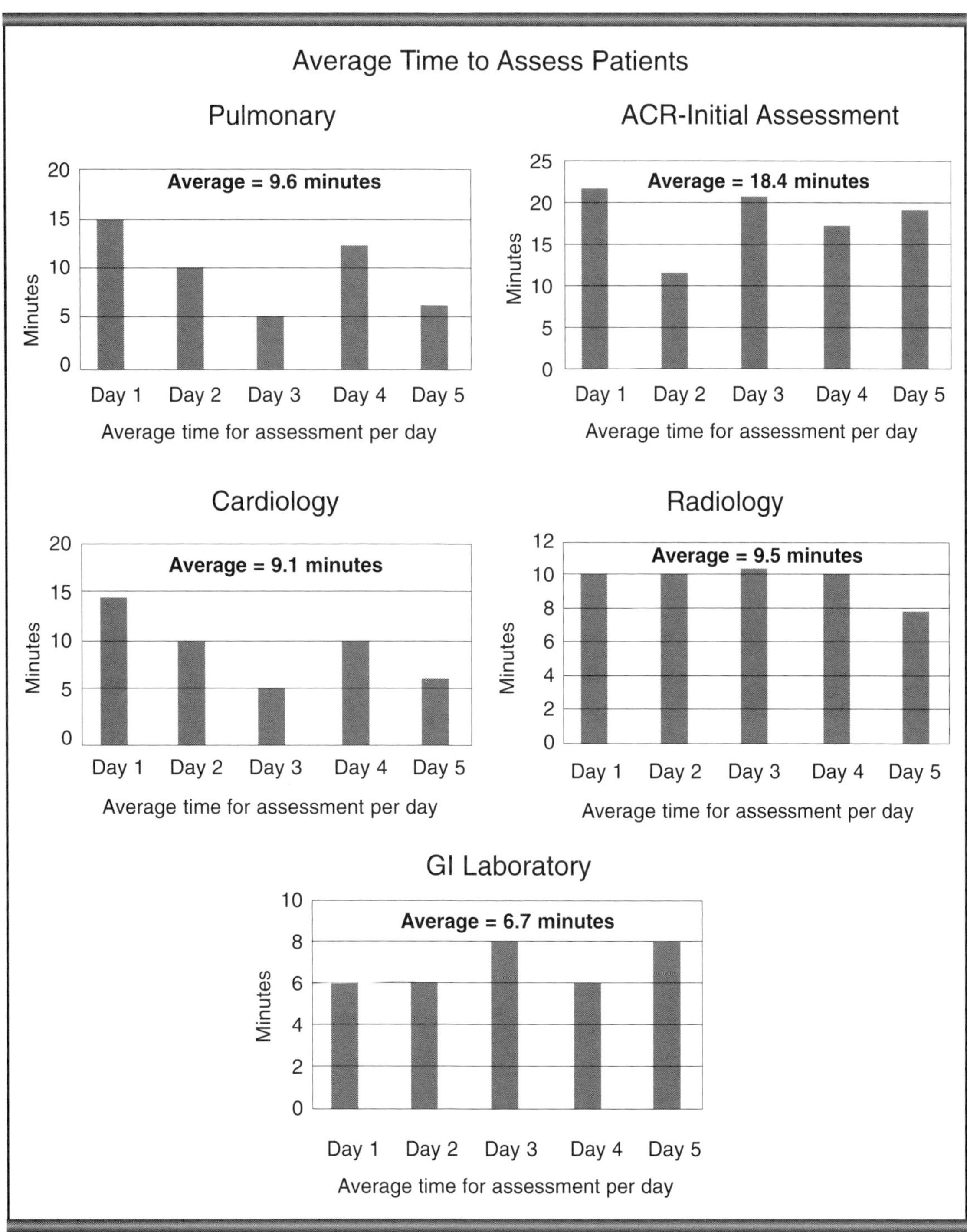

Figure 4-13. The average time it took nurses to gather and document patient assessment information varied from a low of 6.7 minutes in the gastrointestinal laboratory to a high of 18.4 minutes in the ambulatory care recovery unit.
***Source:* Hoag Memorial Hospital Presbyterian, Newport Beach, CA. Used with permission.**

SPECIAL PROCEDURE DATA COLLECTION SHEET

OUTPATIENT ADMISSION

Pt. Name: ________ Date: ______ Time: ______ VS: T___ P ___ R ___ BP __/__
Primary Language: ❑ English ❑ Other: ________ Chief Complaint ________
Planned Procedure: ________ HT: ______ WT: ______ lbs
Advance Directive ❑ Yes ❑ No Decision Maker: ________ ❑ Consents Signed ❑ PT.ID Band on
Family Location/phone #: ________ Discharge care giver: ________ Phone #: ________
Allergies: ❑ No ❑ Yes: ________ Reaction: ________
Diet: ❑ NPO ❑ Clear Liquid ❑ Meal Time: ________ ❑ Isolation ________
❑ Pre Procedure Prep: ❑ Complete ❑ Incomplete ❑ Pre Lab Work: ❑ Pending ❑ On Chart
❑ Prosthesis: ________ Items w/patient: ❑ glasses/contact lens ❑ hearing aid ❑ dentures

NURSING HISTORY AND PHYSICAL

Medical history obtained from ________ Assessed by: ________

Neurological: ❑ Denies Problems ABN ________
Cardiovascular: ❑ Denies Problems ABN ________
Pulmonary: ❑ Denies Problems ABN ________
Gastro Intestinal: ❑ Denies Problems ABN ________
Genitourinary: ❑ Denies Problems ABN ________
Musculoskeletal: ❑ Denies Problems ABN ________
Integumentary: ❑ Denies Problems ABN ________

Meds Taken at home:	Last dose

Other: ❑ Smoker ❑ ETOH Use ❑ Recreational drug use ❑ Hepatitis ❑ Diabetes ❑ TB
Other: ________ Surgeries: ________
Mental/Emotional status: ❑ Calm ❑ Anxious ❑ Fearful ❑ Depressed ❑ Disoriented ❑ Other
Abuse Identified: ❑ Elder ❑ Child ❑ Spouse ❑ Sexual ❑ Emotional ❑ Neglect
Actions Taken:

Prophylatic Meds: ❑ No Pred-Meds ❑ No

Medication	Time	Route

IV: Site: ________ Type/Gauge: ________
Attempts: ________
❑ Good blood return ❑ Site Clear
❑ Hickman ❑ Portacath ❑ Other
❑ Solution: ________
❑ Saline Lock RN Initial ______

❑ INPATIENT ADMISSION ❑ SUBSEQUENT OP ADMISSION - Time:

❑ Verbal ❑ I.D. Band on ❑ Correct Chart ❑ Stamp plate in chart ❑ MAR ❑ Old Chart ❑ ECU Admission Form
Planned Procedure: ________ Reason for Exam: ________ ❑ Consent Signed
❑ Foley cath ❑ Pacemaker ❑ Drain tubes: ________
Diet: ❑ NPO ❑ Liquids ❑ Meal Time: ________ Void Time: ________
IV: Location: ________ ❑ Intact Fluid: #1 ________ #2 ________
❑ Pre Procedure Prep: ❑ Complete ❑ Incomplete ❑ Pre Lab Work: ❑ Pending ❑ On Chart
Items w/patient: ❑ glasses/contact lens ❑ hearing aid ❑ dentures ❑ Family location/phone #: ________
❑ Homework ❑ Hoag Recent (< 2 hours of procedure) Vital Signs: T ___ P ___ R ___ BP ________

❑ INPATIENT ADMISSION ❑ SUBSEQUENT OP ADMISSION - Time:

❑ Verbal ❑ I.D. Band on ❑ Correct Chart ❑ Stamp plate in chart ❑ MAR ❑ Old Chart ❑ ECU Admission Form
Planned Procedure: ________ Reason for Exam: ________ ❑ Consent Signed
❑ Foley cath ❑ Pacemaker ❑ Drain tubes: ________
Diet: ❑ NPO ❑ Liquids ❑ Meal Time: ________ Void Time: ________
IV: Location: ________ ❑ Intact Fluid: #1 ________ #2 ________
❑ Pre Procedure Prep: ❑ Complete ❑ Incomplete ❑ Pre Lab Work: ❑ Pending ❑ On Chart
Items w/ patient: ❑ glasses/contact lens ❑ hearing aid ❑ dentures ❑ Family location/phone #: ________
Recent (< 2 hours of procedure) Vital Signs: T ___ P ___ R ___ BP ________

Continued on page 121.

Figure 4-14. The team condensed the various patient assessment forms used throughout the organization into one 6-page form. This figure shows only two pages of the form. *Source:* Hoag Memorial Hospital Presbyterian, Newport Beach, CA. Used with permission.

Continued from page 120.

Patient Name: ____________________

PULMONARY

Arrival Time: ______ Room: ______ Start Time: ______ Stop Time: ______ Discharge: ______
RCP ______ RN ______ MD ______
Procedure Monitors: ❑ EKG Monitor ❑ Pulse OX ❑ BP ❑ Other: ______

Time	Modality				Duration	Medications	O_2 device/FIO_2
	FFNVIA	❑ MP	❑ Mask	❑ VentMed			
	FIO_2	❑ Air	❑ O_2 @ ______	LPM			

Scope: ______
❑ 1% Lidocaine (Xylocaine) ______ ml
❑ 2% Lidocaine (Xylocaine) ______ ml
❑ 2% Viscous Lidocaine (Xylocaine) ______ ml
❑ 4% Lidocaine (Xylocaine) ______ ml
❑ Epinephrine (1:20,000 Soln) ______ ml
❑ 10% Acetylcysteine (Mucomyst) ______ ml
❑ Other: ______ ______ ml

MEDICATIONS ADMINISTERED BY PHYSICIAN/NURSE: DRUG	CONCENTRATION	ROUTE	AMOUNT GIVEN	AMOUNT WASTED (IF CONTROLLED SUBSTANCE)	PHYSICIAN/NURSE SIGNATURE
Midazolam (versed)	mg/ml		mg	mg	
Flumazenil (Romazicon)	mg/ml		mg	mg	
Other:	mg/ml		mg	mg	

CARDIOVASCULAR

Arrival time: ______ Room: ______ Start Time: ______ Stop Time: ______ Discharge: ______
RN 1 ______ RN 2 ______ TECH 1 ______ TECH 2 ______ MD ______

Treadmill	EKG	NICE	Procedure Code: Cine Film #:	V Access: ______ A Access: ______	Total Heparin ______ mg Total Protamin ______ mg

INTERNAL DEVICES/TREATMENT		Site 1 HEMOSTAsIS	Site 2
❑ Stent ______	❑ Other ______	❑ C clamp ❑ Manual	❑ C clamp ❑ Manual
❑ Pacemaker ______	❑ Tracking documentation completed	Total Time: ______	Total Time: ______
❑ Thrombolysis ______		❑ Hematoma ______ cm	❑ Hematoma ______ cm

ANGIOGRAPHY

Arrival Time: ______ Room: ______ Start Time: ______ Stop Time: ______ Discharge: ______
RN 1 ______ RN 2 ______ TECH 1 ______ TECH 2 ______ MD ______

Pulse Pre/Post	RDP	RPT	LDP	LPT	R/L Brachial	R/L Radial	Total Heparin ______ mg
	/	/	/	/	/	/	Total Protamine ______ mg

(1) Access: ______ ❑ Sheath ______ ❑ Catheter ______ ❑ Wire ______ ❑ DC'D: ______
(2) Access: ______ ❑ Sheath ______ ❑ Catheter ______ ❑ Wire ______ ❑ DC'D: ______

INTERNAL DEVICES/TREATMENT		Site 1 HEMOSTASIS	Site 2
❑ Stent ______	❑ Coil ______	❑ C clamp ❑ Manual	❑ C clamp ❑ Manual
❑ Filter ______	❑ Embolic Mat. ______	Total Time: ______	Total time: ______
❑ Thrombolysis	❑ Tracking documentation completed	❑ Hematoma ______ cm	Hematoma ______ cm

GI LAB

Arrival Time: ______ Room: ______ Start Time: ______ Stop Time: ______ Discharge: ______
Initial sedation by: ______ MD: ______ RN: ______ 2nd Assist: ______
Scope Number: ______ Scope: GIF __/__ CF __/__ JF __/__ Other: __/__
Inserted by: ______ Into: Esophagus/rectum/Ostomy Advanced by: ______ To: Duodenum/Cecum/Other ______
Treatment: ❑ pH ❑ Photos ❑ Sclerotherapy ______ cc SOLN ❑ ERCP ❑ Biopsy ❑ Cytology ❑ CLO Test
❑ Polypectomy ______ Settings ______ ❑ Dilation-type ______ FR ______
❑ Bicap ______ Settings ______ ❑ Grounding Pad: Location ______
❑ Sphincterotomy-equip ______ Settings ______ Lot No: ______
❑ Peg-brand ______ Lot No. ______ FR ______ Length ______
❑ Stent placement-equip ______ FR ______ Length ______ ❑ Scope Out Time: ______ ❑ Airway maintained
❑ EGD ❑ Colonoscopy ❑ ECRP ❑ Other ______ ❑ Ground pad skin site intact-post procedure

OTHER

Examination:
R.N. 1 ______ R.N. 2 ______ Tech 1 ______ Tech 2 ______ M.D. ______
Arrival Time: ______ Room: ______ Start Time: ______ Stop Time: ______ Discharge: ______

Initials	Signature/Title

Addressograph

The Next Step

The team set up performance measures to monitor the efficiency and satisfaction of the new patient assessment form. In one such measurement activity, the team decided to measure how long it would take procedure nurses to complete their patient assessments with the new form. The team expected that it should only take 2 to 3 minutes for nurses to complete the form versus the 10 to 15 minutes they had previously spent. The team also planned to interview patients regarding their satisfaction with the new process.

Example 4-3. Benchmarking Asthma Care in a Public Health Agency

The Setting and Background

Lincoln County Community Health Center is a hypothetical government agency that manages five public health clinics and two school-based centers. These health centers provide primary care to the low-income population in a hypothetical county of Arizona.

The agency has been using quality improvement techniques for the last several years. Multidisciplinary teams have improved patient waiting times, medication dispensing, and other administrative processes. This year, agency leaders decide to focus on improving clinical processes. They begin by identifying the patient populations or medical conditions that are high volume, high cost, and problem prone. They identify six clinical areas:

- Asthma;
- Heart disease;
- Diabetes;
- Depression;
- Low back pain; and
- Childhood immunizations.

Example Highlights

Setting:
Lincoln County Community Health Center

Performance Improvement Initiative:
Develop a process to improve assessment and treatment of patients with asthma across multiple settings

Dimensions of Performance Addressed:
Appropriateness, availability, continuity, effectiveness, efficacy, efficiency, safety, timeliness.

Comments:
This example illustrates how an interdisciplinary team uses benchmarking to identify a need for improvement.

Leaders assign a task force to oversee clinical improvement projects in each of these areas. The teams are asked to identify the best ways to manage these conditions across the continuum, including disease prevention, proper assessment, and treatment.

Assessing Asthma Care

The asthma care task force includes two primary care physicians, two nurses, and a respiratory therapist. Task force members begin by reviewing data on the asthma population at the agency's various clinics (for example, number of patients, age).

Then the team makes a flowchart of the process used to assess and treat asthma patients. They find that this process varies from physician to physician and from clinic to clinic. They highlight those areas of the process that contain a lot of variation.

See page 104 for a discussion on flowcharts.

The task force then gathers outcomes data from the last three years on the number of asthma patients with emergency room and inpatient admissions. After reviewing the literature, they find that the agency's rate is above the national average.

Benchmarking Asthma Care

Through a literature review, the team identifies several primary care clinics that have significantly improved outcomes for asthma patients. The two nurses call and interview staff in each of these organizations to learn what processes they follow.

In addition, the team identifies an internal benchmark. By stratifying outcomes data by clinic and by physician, the team finds that one of the agency's clinics has a significantly lower emergency room and inpatient admission rate for asthma patients. The nurse manager of that clinic attends one of the team's meetings and describes how they manage asthma patients. Based on this research, the team identifies several best practices for asthma management:

- Regularly scheduled visits with primary care physician;
- Educational sessions that teach asthmatics how to use inhalers and proper use of anti-inflammatory drugs; and
- Home visits by a home care nurse or nurse case manager to assess the home environment and provide follow-up care.

Implementing Improvements

The team develops a clinical protocol for asthma assessment and treatment that incorporates all of these best practices. On diagnosis, all asthma patients now meet one-on-one with a nurse educator. In addition, a community nurse case manager visits the patient's home, at their convenience, to assess the home environment for possible irritants (for example, pets).

To implement the new protocol, the team holds several meetings with clinic staff to educate them about the new procedure and launches a communications campaign, which includes posters and articles in the clinic newsletter, to remind staff to follow the new protocol.

Three months later, the agency's rate of emergency room and inpatient admissions for asthma drops by 45%. When team members review the data, they find that most of the asthma patients currently being admitted to the hospital are children. As a result, the team is currently designing a education program specifically for parents of asthmatic children.

References

Camp RC: *Benchmarking: The Search for Industry Best Practices That Lead To Superior Performance.* Milwaukee, WI: American Society for Quality Control (ASQC) Quality Press, 16–21, 1989.

Flower J: *Springboard or Buzzword?* Joint Commission Health Care Forum, Jan-Feb 1993.

Using Performance Improvement Tools in Health Care Settings. Oakbrook Terrace, IL; Joint Commission on Accreditation of Healthcare Organizations, 1996.

CHAPTER 5: Improve

Chapter Highlights

What Are the Goals of Improvement?

- Continued improvement, not "optimal" performance;
- Specific, measurable improvements for identified dimensions of performance;
- Improvements that are measurable and sustained; and
- Improvements that target processes but address any issues associated with individual clinicians or staff.

Who Takes Improvement Actions?

- The process' owners, customers, and suppliers design and test improvements.
- The organization's leaders approve changes that involve significant resources or effects.
- Changes should be explained in an educational, non-threatening way to all people who carry out the process.

Continued on page 126.

Continued from page 125.

How Do We Improve Processes?

- Use a systematic method to plan, test, assess, and fully implement the changes;
- Use qualitative and quantitative tools, including multivoting, selection grids, cause-and-effect diagrams, run charts, flowcharts, and histograms; and
- Use critical paths to design new processes, redesign existing processes, monitor health outcomes, and evaluate cost effectiveness of care.

Examples of Improvement

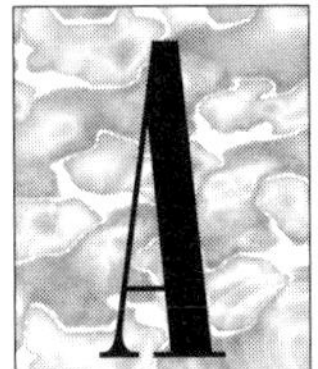

mbulatory care organizations are rapidly realizing that the world of health care has dramatically changed. Ambulatory care organizations must be able to compete to survive and prosper.

The fundamental outcome of the framework for improving performance is improvement. Taken together, design, measurement, and assessment culminate in specific actions to improve performance. Improvements come about through redesign of existing processes or through innovation and design of new processes. Figure 5-1, below, shows the relationship of this phase to the rest of the cycle for improving performance.

What Are the Goals of Improvement?

Improvement is a continuous process. The following questions will help organizations set goals and develop a comprehensive plan for their improvement efforts.

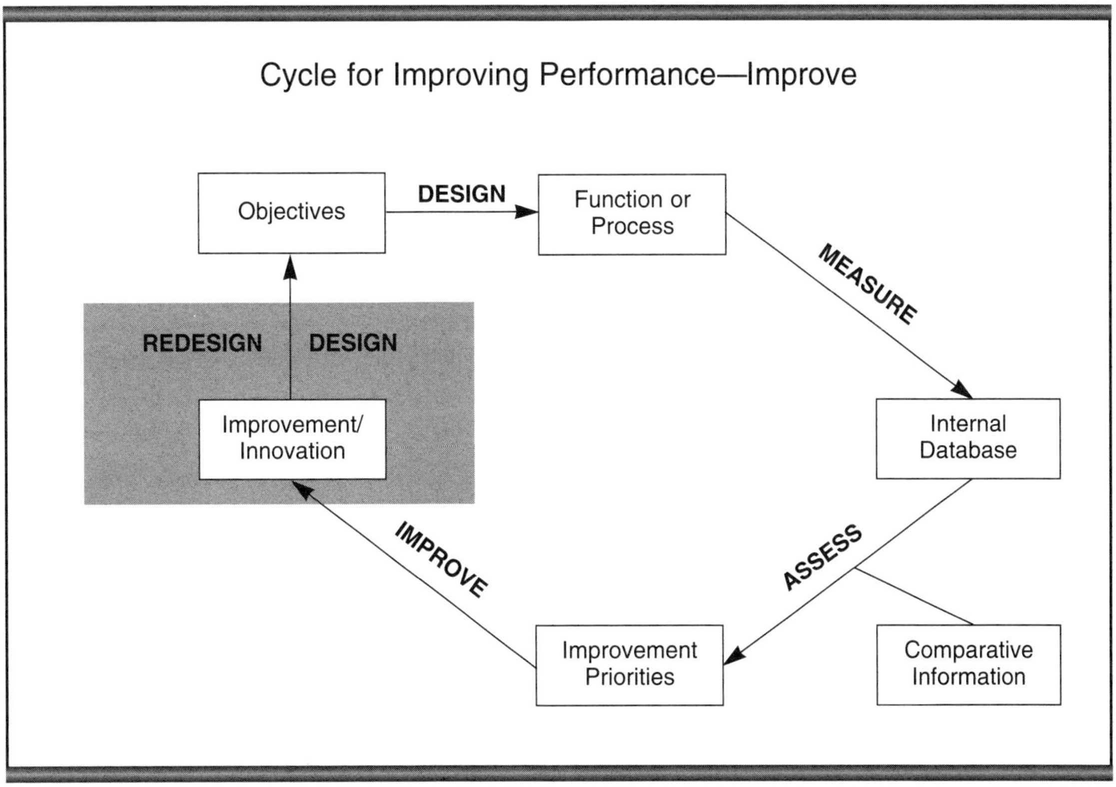

Cycle for Improving Performance—Improve

Objectives
DESIGN
Function or Process
MEASURE
Internal Database
ASSESS
Comparative Information
Improvement Priorities
IMPROVE
Improvement/ Innovation
REDESIGN
DESIGN

Figure 5-1. By adding improve and redesign/design, the cycle is complete.

What dimension(s) of performance will be most affected by the change? To understand the potential effects of the improvement activity, the organization must determine which dimensions of performance will be affected. At times, the relationship between two or more dimensions must be considered. For example, when a service's availability is increased, the process's efficiency may decline, but cost per unit of service may decrease. As mentioned in Chapter 2, this understanding of goals for improvement will also be affected by the type and nature of the care delivered. For example, how does care delivered in an imaging center differ from treatment delivered in a community health center? How are the dimensions of performance organized in each care environment?

How do we expect, want, and need the improved process to perform? The ambulatory care organization and the team carrying out the effort should set specific expectations for performance resulting from the design or improvement process (for example, patient waiting time will decrease by 20%). These expectations can be derived from staff expertise, patient/public expectations, experiences of other organizations, recognized standards, and other sources. Without these performance expectations, the organization will not be able to determine the degree of success of the efforts or judge its improvements overall.

How will we measure to determine if the process is actually performing at the level we expect? The organization and team will need specific tools to measure the performance of the newly designed or improved process to determine whether performance expectations are met. These measures can be borrowed or adapted from other sources, or they can be newly created, as appropriate. As always, the measurement will be subject to the traditional guidelines of the scientific method.

Who is closest to this process and therefore should "own" a portion of the improvement activity? To a great extent, the success of an improvement effort hinges on involving the right people from all disciplines, services, and offices involved in the process being addressed. For example, an effort to improve continuity of care for a community health center might involve appropriate representatives from nursing, social work, case management, and administration, as well as physicians and patients. For example, a life safety project in an endoscopy center might include clinicians, nursing staff, and a life safety expert.

Processes and Individuals

Improvement actions should be directed primarily at processes. As stated earlier in this book, process improvement holds the greatest opportunity for significant change, whereas changes related to an individual's performance may have limited effect. As in many endeavors, good people often find themselves carrying out bad processes.

Individual performance cannot, however, be ignored. The possible consequences of skill, knowledge, or judgment problems are grave, sometimes life threatening. Therefore, when measurement and assessment direct attention to an individual's performance, appropriate action must be taken. This action often takes the form of counseling, education, or activity restriction. In the occasional cases in which care professionals cannot or will not address performance problems, other actions are necessary in accordance with policies and procedures, such as modifying their job assignments or scope of responsibilities.

Who Takes Improvement Actions?

As with other phases of the improvement cycle, involving the right people from the beginning is essential. Leaders should make every effort to involve all staff who carry out and have knowledge of the process or function being improved, including physicians, nurses, and administrative staff. Equally important is patient feedback. The process for taking action consists of several stages, each of which may have different players and teams.

Designing the Action

In general, the group that has measured and assessed the process should have the necessary expertise to recommend improvements and is in the best position to design the improvements. This group should include those who carry out and are affected by the process. The group may also ask staff with special expertise to serve as consultants on an as-needed basis in the design or evaluation process.

Approving Recommended Actions

When substantial resources are involved and the potential effects are significant, the organization's leaders will usually become involved in reviewing and approving the action. For instance, if a team determines that the best way to streamline the client registration process is to purchase a new information system, then leaders will want to carefully consider the financial implications of such a change.

In other cases, a solution may be relatively simple to implement (for example, shifting duties within a service area, or changing a minor aspect of an existing process). Such a change usually can be approved by the appropriate manager. Final approval should come more readily if a team obtains the necessary input and buy-in while devising the improvement.

Testing the Action

Before implementing any improvement, the team should conduct a pilot test to ensure that the change results in an actual improvement. Testing should occur under "real world" conditions, involving staff who will actually be carrying out the process under day-to-day operations. For example, a clinic that wants to test out a new appointment process might pilot the process on patients whose last names begin with A–D for three months. The results can be measured with the same methods used to establish a performance baseline.

Implementing the Action

After careful piloting, full-scale implementation of a process change should have significant and positive results. However, any change can create anxiety. Therefore, care should be taken to prepare staff and clients for change and to explain the reason for the change in an educational, nonthreatening way. Holding in-services or brown bag lunches to explain the change in process or placing notices on clinic bulletin boards and in newsletters are two possible approaches.

Cooperation is viewed as essential for changes to succeed, and typically will not occur if people believe a change is being forced on them. An effective team should have already acquired much of the necessary buy-in during earlier phases of the improvement process. Appendix B, page 193, provides further suggestions for promoting effective teamwork in implementing improvement initiatives and highlights a model of progress for a project team.

How Do We Improve Processes? Tools and Methods for Improvement and Innovation

Once the goals and priorities for improvement have been established, the organization can begin planning and carrying out innovations. A standard, yet flexible, process for carrying out these changes should help leaders and others to ensure that process improvement actions address root causes, involve appropriate people, result in desired and sustained changes, and ultimately improve outcomes. The fundamental components of any improvement process include:

- Defining the problem/opportunity for change;
- Testing the change;
- Studying its effects; and
- Implementing changes determined to be worthwhile.

The Scientific Method

Many readers will readily associate the activities listed above with the basic scientific method. Indeed, the scientific method is the fundamental, inclusive paradigm for change, and includes the following:

1) Determine what we know now (about a process, problem, topic of interest).
2) Decide what we want to learn, change, or improve.
3) Develop a hypothesis about how the change can be accomplished.
4) Test the hypothesis.
5) Assess the effect of the test. Compare results "before versus after" or "traditional versus innovative."
6) Implement successful improvements or rehypothesize and conduct another experiment.
7) Generalize the innovation to all relevant areas.

This orderly, logical, inclusive process for improvement will serve health care organizations well as they assess and improve performance.

Plan-Do-Check-Act

A well-established process for improvement that is based on the scientific method is the plan-do-check-act (PDCA) cycle (see Figure 5-2, page 132). This process is attributed to Walter Shewhart, a quality improvement pioneer and is

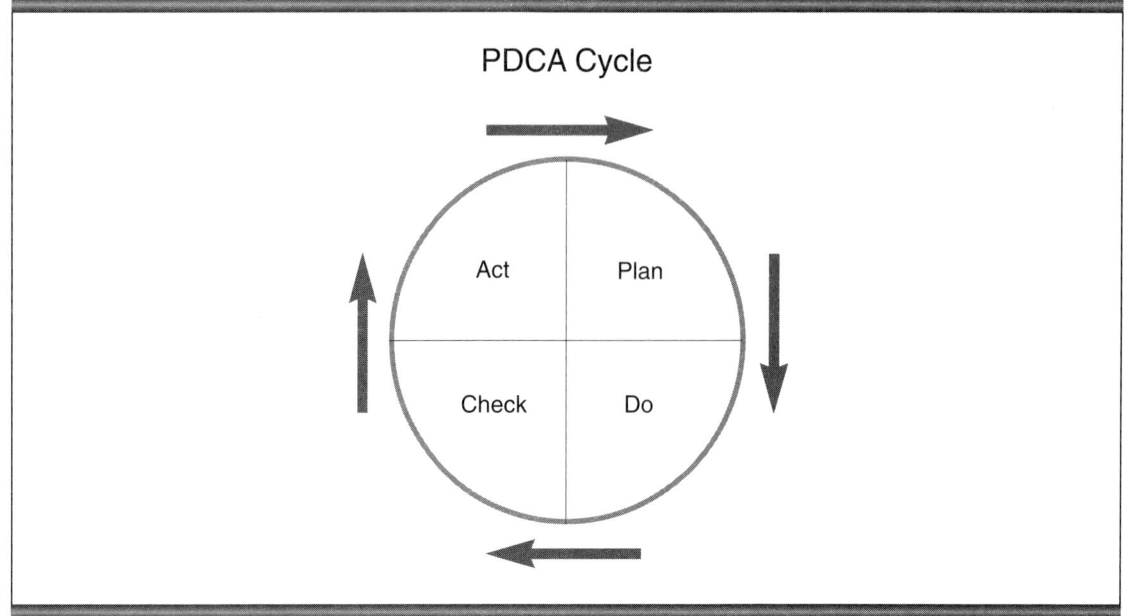

Figure 5-2. The PDCA cycle is useful in planning, testing, assessing, and implementing an action to improve a process.

widely associated with W. Edwards Deming, a student and later a colleague of Shewhart. A summary of the PDCA cycle is provided in Table 5-1, page 133.

Plan. During this step, an operational plan for testing the chosen improvement action is created. Small-scale testing or pilot testing is necessary to determine whether the improvement actions are viable, whether they will have the desired result, and whether any refinements are necessary before putting them into full operation. The list of proposed improvement actions should be narrowed to a number that can be reasonably tested—seldom more than two to four improvement actions.

During the planning stage, several issues should be resolved:

- Why is the idea being tested?
- Who will be involved in the test?
- What do they need to know to participate in the test?
- What are the testing timetables?
- How will the test be implemented?
- What are the success factors?
- How will the process and outcomes of the test be measured and assessed?

Table 5-1. Key Steps of the PDCA Cycle.

Plan:

- Determine data needed to monitor the improvement in the process.
- Determine tests for the improvement monitoring plan.

Do:

- Collect and analyze data on improvement in the process.
- Make improvement changes/actions when indicated and appropriate.

Check:

- Establish decision/review points to determine the effectiveness of changes.
- Assess the effects of improvements.
- Analyze the improvement results.

Act:

- Team meets on a regular basis to determine what was learned.
- Tests or actions are repeated, if necessary, to ensure improvement in the process.
- Generalized improvements.

Do. This step involves implementing the pilot test and collecting actual performance data.

Check. The data collected during the pilot test are analyzed to determine whether the improvement action was successful in achieving the desired outcome(s). To determine the degree of success, actual test performance is compared to desired performance targets and baseline results achieved using the established process.

Act. The next step is to take action. If the pilot test is not successful, the cycle is repeated. Once actions have been shown to be successful, they are made part of standard operating procedure.

The process does not stop here, though. In the future, the effectiveness of the action will continue to be measured and assessed to ensure that improvement is maintained.

Critical Paths

One significant improvement method not yet discussed is the critical path (also referred to as the clinical path, critical or clinical pathway, and practice parameter or guideline).* Several factors have converged to spur the development of critical paths, including: ongoing cost containment forces; total quality management initiatives to reduce practice variation; and emergence of consistent and reliable treatment approaches. Critical paths offer a systematic, flexible guide for patient care. They include descriptions of acceptable methods to diagnose, manage, treat, or prevent specific diseases and conditions.

Such guides can be used by physicians, nurses, and other staff to guide—but not mandate—the care delivery process. They are designed by those involved in the process—nurses, physicians, and others—who come together to offer their unique perspectives and expertise. It is important to note that guidelines must be seen as a dynamic process that incorporates ongoing development and outcome assessments with practice updates and revision.

A critical path is an excellent way to approach the design of the process for a new service or a complete redesign for an existing process that needs change. One advantage of a critical path is the opportunity to start fresh, cast aside traditional but not particularly effective procedures, and research and implement the best practices.

Selecting the process. The initial step in creating a critical path is choosing a process to standardize. Ambulatory care organizations perform a wide range of diagnoses and procedures, treat a variety of conditions, and offer many different services. Likely candidates for redesign will be processes that are high volume, high risk, problem prone, costly, important to staff or patients, vital to the organization's mission, or that represent a cross-discipline, cross-functional process.

---

*While these terms are often used interchangeably, there are some differences. The terms are all included under a definition of practice protocols; *critical pathways* are a treatment regime, with consensus of clinicians that include only a few elements proven to affect patient outcomes; *clinical pathways* are similar, but broader and include all elements of care; *practice parameters* represent an agreed upon strategy for patient management deemed acceptable practice by professional organizations. (*Hospital Risk Management* 16(2):20, Feb 1994)

Defining the boundaries of the path. The critical path can begin anytime during the episode of care, such as patient diagnosis or initial assessment. For example, an integrated critical pathway can follow a patient across various health care settings.

Defining the diagnosis, condition, or procedure. An appropriately defined process and patient population to be served will simplify critical path development. Identify as clearly and precisely as possible the patient population for whom the path is designed. A process that is too broadly defined will result in a path that is either too complex or too vague; conversely, a process that is too narrowly defined can result in a path that applies to only a limited number of cases. For example, an ambulatory care organization may begin its critical path development by defining the most frequent patient diagnoses served in the previous year and studying approaches to assessment and treatment in this group (for example, all diabetic patients).

Forming a path design team. The group that creates the critical path must represent all disciplines involved in the process. For example, a team developing a critical path for asthma management would likely include nurses, physicians, pharmacists, respiratory therapists, and others. Another valuable perspective comes from patients and their families or care givers. The team should elicit information from the people the process is designed to benefit and from other involved parties.

Creating the critical path. To progress, team members will need to reach consensus on the key activities involved in each stage of the care process. Members can draw on personal experience and knowledge, existing clinical literature and practice guidelines, and patient perspectives. Be assured that varying styles, methods, and approaches to care will arise in the team review. The resulting discussion can yield important knowledge about care delivery. If varied practice patterns are such that the group cannot reach consensus, the path should not dictate one approach over the other. Over time, the value of various critical paths can be evaluated empirically.

Remember also that the path need not be limited to clinical activities. For example, a critical path might address the process used to dispense medications to patients or make patient appointments. Critical paths should also include outcomes.

Despite the complexity of the processes involved, teams should attempt to make their paths as concise as possible—one page is ideal—so they can be used as practical tools in daily practice.

The time needed to develop a critical path may vary from two hours to one year. Organizations should be prepared to invest a significant commitment of time and effort during the development cycle.

Typically, critical paths will address many specific areas of care including:

- Consultations;
- Diagnostic testing;
- Medications;
- Treatments/interventions;
- Nutrition;
- Education;
- Symptom control;
- Health education;
- Prevention;
- Wellness;
- Self-treatment options;
- Alternative treatment options; and
- Expected outcomes.

Defining the care delivery outcomes that are expected during the episode of care covered by the critical path. Outcomes have become an increasingly important aspect of all patient-focused management activities. This perspective is reflected in critical path development. The critical path design team determines what the patient is expected to achieve or be able to perform at specific intervals in the care plan.

Results. At all stages of the care process, staff, especially clinical staff, can refer to critical paths to guide decision making. They should be available to all involved personnel in all the relevant work areas and office locations. Critical paths are also valuable for patients; they can increase patients' knowledge of the care plan and sense of partnership with providers.

Examples of Improvement

Example 5-1. Improving Patient Education Documentation at a Correctional Facility

The Setting and Background

The Tucson Federal Correctional Institution is a medium-level security facility that houses inmates sentenced to a federal facility, pre-trial male inmates, and pre-trial/holdover female inmates. The population shifts on a daily basis; currently, there are approximately 825 inmates. During an average day, a total of 60 or more patients are seen.

The Problem

In May 1995, health services staff conducted a continuous quality improvement (CQI) study to determine the department's compliance with a Bureau of Prison policy related to chronic care in specialty clinics. One criterion in this policy is that patient education should be provided to all chronic care patients and then should be documented in the medical record. To determine how well the department complied with this criterion, staff reviewed 18 records. From this retrospective review, staff learned that only 22%, or 4 of the 18 records, contained documentation that patient education was provided during chronic care visits. Department staff were concerned that patients were either not receiving education on chronic diseases or that care givers were not documenting the education they provided in the record.

Health services staff believed that the purpose of education was to promote positive health outcomes for inmates while they are incarcerated and when they are released to the community. The increased number and age of inmates, coupled with the current rise in health care costs and cutbacks in government spending,

Example Highlights

Setting:
Tucson Federal Correctional Institution, Tucson, Arizona

Performance Improvement Initiative:
Improve the frequency and documentation of patient education.

Dimensions of Performance Addressed:
Availability, continuity, effectiveness, efficacy, efficiency, timeliness.

Comments:
This example illustrates how a quality improvement team identifies a need for improvement, designs and implements a plan, and monitors progress.

made patient education a critical mandate for health care providers in correctional facilities.

The Team

The department's CQI and Risk Management Committee met monthly and consisted of the chief physician, a health services administrator, an assistant health services administrator, a registered nurse, a certified family nurse practitioner, physician assistants, dentists, an accredited record technician, a medical secretary, and a dental assistant. Staff reported the findings of the above CQI study to the committee.

The Process

The committee identified and implemented the following corrective actions:

- The clinical coordinator developed health teaching fact cards covering such topics as hypertension, diabetes, asthma, and exercises for a healthy heart. The brochures were printed in both English and Spanish and distributed to all clinical providers.
- The chief physician was provided with a stamp stating "Patient given handout on *(specific medical problem)*." The stamp served as a useful reminder to the physician to provide education when evaluating patients.
- At morning rounds, supervisory staff encouraged and supported patient education.
- While patients were waiting for their appointments, health education videos in English and Spanish were continuously presented.
- Health education brochures were maintained in the waiting room and dental area, covering a broad range of subjects and were made available for inmates in both English and Spanish.

Results and Outcomes

Staff conducted a follow-up CQI study in October 1995. They reviewed the records of 17 inmates who are enrolled in chronic care clinics. Staff found that 94%, or 16 of the 17 records reviewed, contained appropriate documentation of patient education. These findings demonstrated a 72% improvement rate within a five-month period (see Figure 5-3, page 139).

See page 103 for a discussion on histograms.

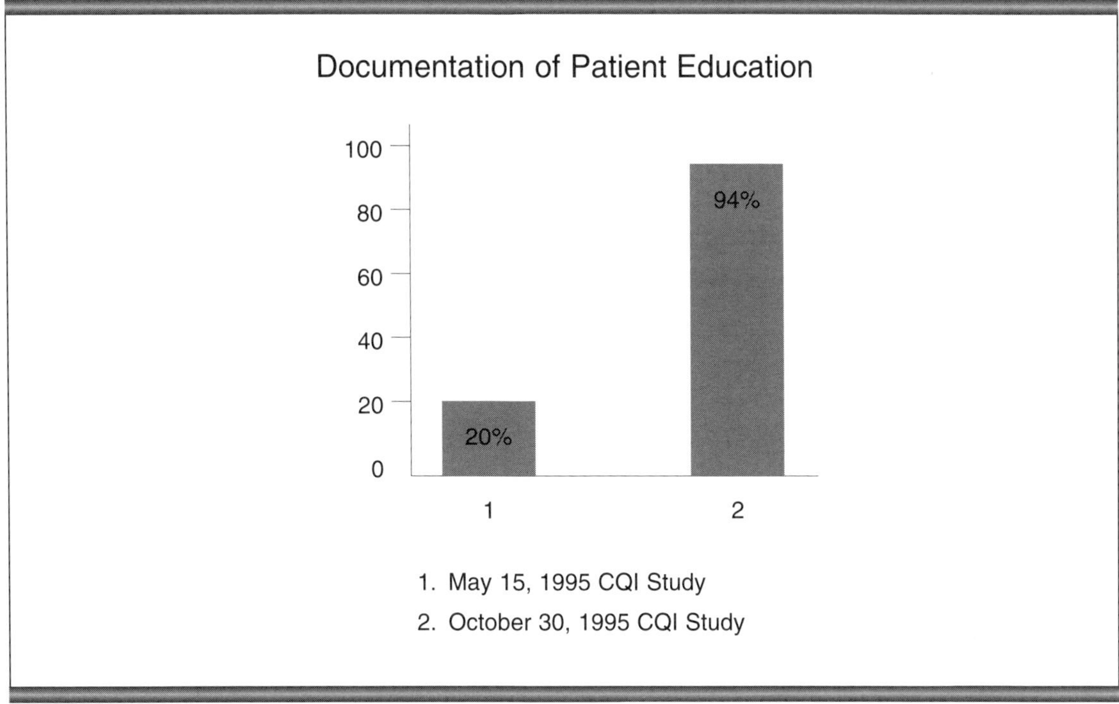

Figure 5-3. After implementing several improvements, the number of patient records that appropriately documented patient education increased by 72%.
Source: **Tucson Federal Correctional Institution, Tucson, AZ. Used with permission.**

Ultimately, the department's goal was 100% compliance. Currently, patient education is being monitored in three ways:

- Medical audits conducted monthly by the accredited record technician and reported to health services staff;
- Regular CQI studies conducted by the CQI Coordinator and the certified family nurse practitioner; and
- Random chart audits conducted by the physician assistant on morning watch.

The results will be reported to the CQI and Risk Management Committee. In addition, the department has implemented a health promotion and disease prevention program for designated and pre-release inmates. On completion of the course, individuals receive a certificate of completion that is placed in their file.

Example 5-2. Improving Communication in the Preoperative Process at a Surgery Center

The Setting and Background

Built in 1978 to serve Leon County and the surrounding referral areas in Florida, the Tallahassee Single Day Surgery Center is owned by a group of 43 surgeons. It has four operating rooms and 12 recovery beds. The center sees approximately 4,500 patients a year and offers seven specialties: gynecology, urology, ENT, general surgery, ophthalmology, plastic surgery, podiatry, and orthopedics.

To help staff carry out improvement activities, the surgery center has adopted the FOCUS-PDCA problem-solving technique. The quality improvement director developed a questionnaire outlining the FOCUS-PDCA process in language that staff could quickly understand and use. Staff now have a simple step-by-step questionnaire that they can use when trying to improve a particular area (see Figure 5-4, page 141).

Example Highlights

Setting:
Tallahassee Single Day Surgery Center, Tallahassee, Florida

Performance Improvement Initiative:
Streamline the preoperative interview process.

Dimensions of Performance Addressed:
Availability, continuity, efficiency, timeliness.

Comments:
This example illustrates how an interdisciplinary team uses the FOCUS-PDCA problem solving technique with performance improvement tools.

Find a Process to Improve

One of the first areas that the surgery center decided to improve was the preoperative process. In 1993, patients were complaining of 1- to 2-hour waiting times for their preoperative interview or they felt they got lost in the shuffle. The quality improvement director was also receiving many complaints from staff.

Part of the surgery center's mission is to make surgery as pleasant an experience as possible. The lack of communication between the business and nursing areas ran counter to this mission. By improving the preoperative process, managers

Quality Improvement Study

1. What is the opportunity for improvement?

   A. How do you know that there is an opportunity for improvement? (list reasons)
      1.
      2.
      3.
      4.
      5.

   B. Why is it important to staff and/or patient care?

   C. What would you like to see happen?

2A. What is the present way of doing things? (draw and label the steps)
   B. What are the major conditions that affect the every day process?

3A. What are the possible causes of the issue?

   B. What are the more likely causes of the issue?

4. Find an answer/brainstorm.
   A. List ideas (all ideas, no matter how silly).

   B. What is the best answer or most agreed upon solution to the issue?

5. What is your plan?
   A. Fill out the Opportunity Statement Form.
   B. Decide exactly what part of the process you are going to change.
   C. Decide who is going to do what, when, and where.

6. Gather information.
   A. Did you get the result that you wanted?
      1. IF SO, how are you going to make the change permanent?

      2. IF NOT, review your study. Are there other areas of the process that you need to look at?

         a. What is your plan?

Figure 5-4. Staff at Tallahassee Single Day Surgery Center use this simple step-by-step questionnaire when improving a process.
Source: **Tallahassee Single Day Surgery Center, Tallahassee, FL. Used with permission.**

hoped to improve patient satisfaction, decrease stress between work units, enhance public relations, and improve the quality of care.

Organize to Improve the Process

The managers decided to work on this problem themselves. It presented an opportunity for them to learn about quality improvement and the FOCUS-PDCA method. Team members included the executive director, the director of nursing, a clinical supervisor, the quality improvement coordinator, an operating room supervisor, and the business office manager.

Because the managers may have become defensive about this issue and protective of their own turfs, the team set some ground rules that included:

- Be honest;
- No personal attacks or blaming;
- Don't be defensive;
- Be goal-directed or goal-oriented;
- Listen, listen, listen;
- Be open and receptive;
- Use stress management strategy; and
- Be patient.

The team then developed a timeline for solving the preoperative problem (see Figure 5-5, page 143).

Clarify Current Knowledge of the Process

Team members began by developing a flowchart of the current process (see Figure 5-6, page 144).

See page 104 for a discussion on flowcharts.

As they made a flowchart of the process, the managers identified a simple problem that they could correct immediately. Neither nursing nor the business office kept a list of the patients who arrived for their preoperative visit. As a result, staff did not know which patients had arrived or where they were. To solve this problem, the team asked front desk staff to begin making a list of all preoperative patients, including the time they arrived and the time the nurse brought them back for their preoperative interview.

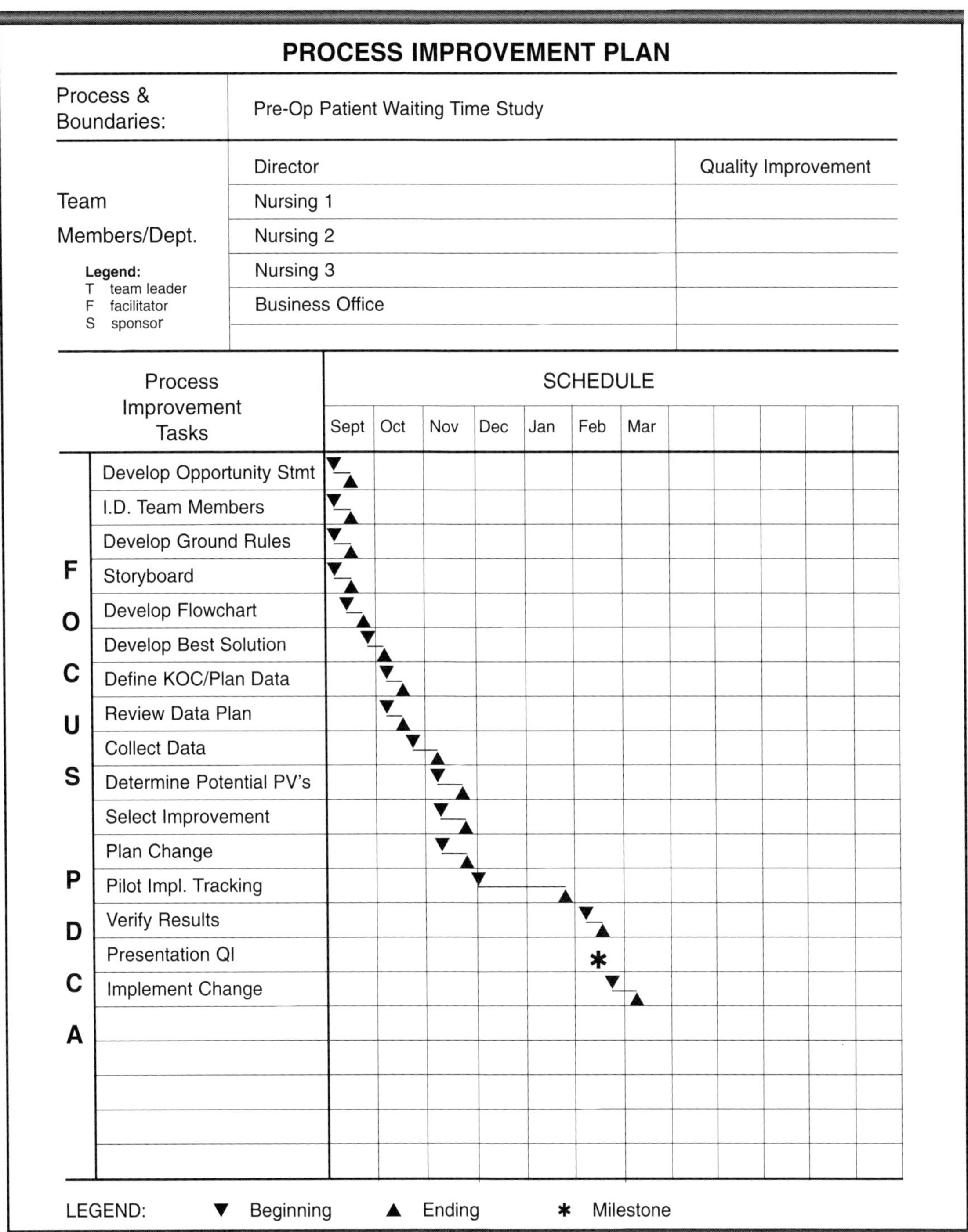

PROCESS IMPROVEMENT PLAN

Process & Boundaries:	Pre-Op Patient Waiting Time Study	
Team Members/Dept.	Director	Quality Improvement
	Nursing 1	
	Nursing 2	
	Nursing 3	
	Business Office	

Legend:
T team leader
F facilitator
S sponsor

	Process Improvement Tasks	Sept	Oct	Nov	Dec	Jan	Feb	Mar					
	Develop Opportunity Stmt	▼ ▲											
	I.D. Team Members	▼ ▲											
	Develop Ground Rules	▼ ▲											
F	Storyboard	▼ ▲											
O	Develop Flowchart	▼ ▲											
	Develop Best Solution	▼	▲										
C	Define KOC/Plan Data		▼ ▲										
U	Review Data Plan		▼ ▲										
	Collect Data		▼	▲									
S	Determine Potential PV's			▼ ▲									
	Select Improvement			▼ ▲									
	Plan Change			▼ ▲									
P	Pilot Impl. Tracking				▼	▲							
D	Verify Results						▼ ▲						
	Presentation QI						✱						
C	Implement Change						▼	▲					
A													

LEGEND: ▼ Beginning ▲ Ending ✱ Milestone

Figure 5-5. Team members developed a time line for the improvement process.
Source: **Tallahassee Single Day Surgery Center, Tallahassee, FL. Used with permission.**

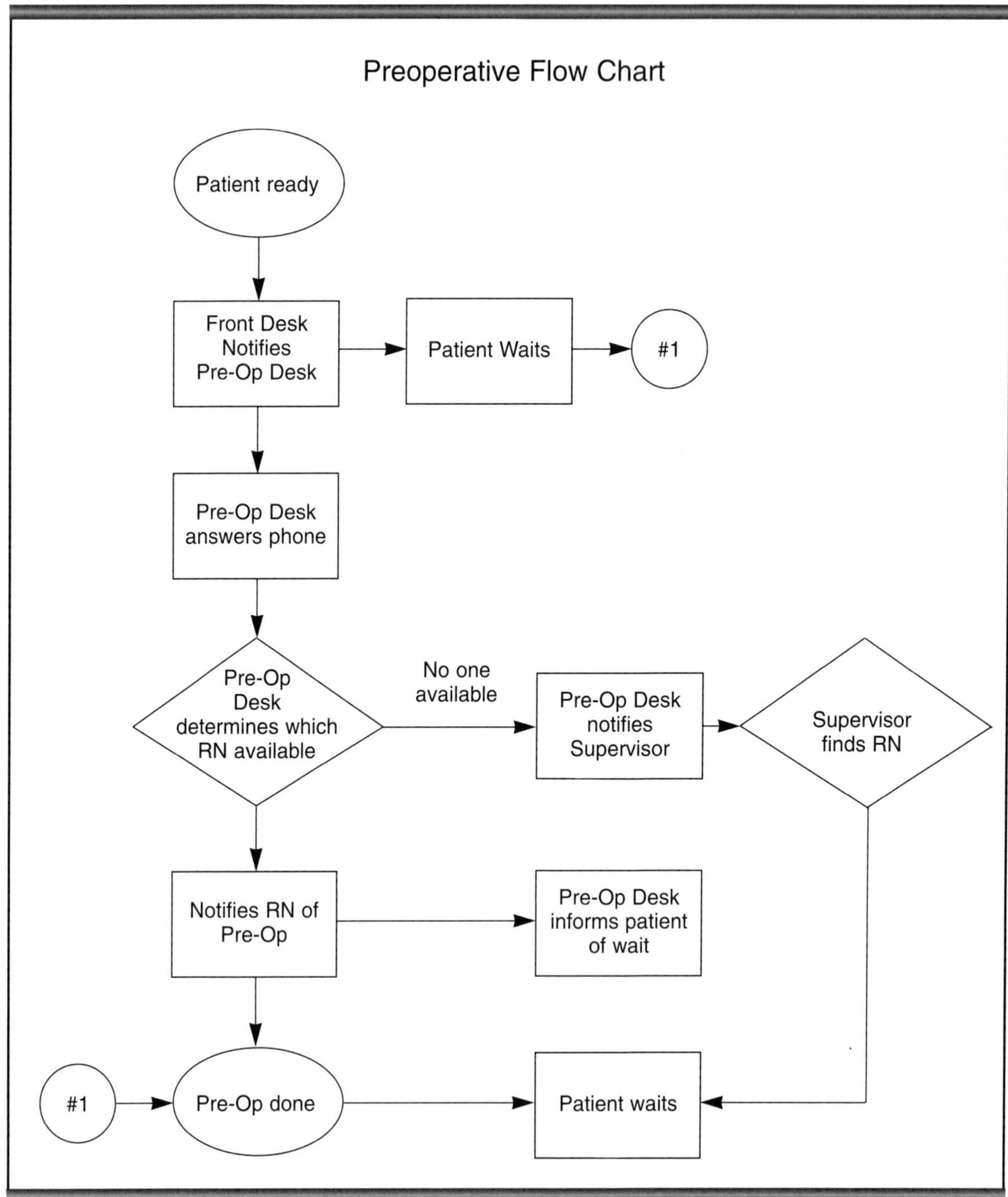

Figure 5-6. Team members developed a flowchart of the preoperative process.
***Source:* Tallahassee Single Day Surgery Center, Tallahassee, FL. Used with permission.**

Understanding Sources of Process Variation

See page 105 for a discussion on cause-and-effect diagrams.

The team brainstormed sources of delays in the preoperative process and placed them in a cause-and-effect diagram. (see Figure 5-7, page 146). Sources of variation included the following:

- Patients do not arrive on time.
- Preoperative delays depended on other preoperative appointments being completed on time.
- Lack of continuity between anesthesiologists, causing delays.
- Nonstandardized preoperative visits.
- Registered nurses will sign off preoperative visits at the preoperative desk before actually going to the patient. Therefore, the desk believes that the patient is being seen when actually he or she is not.
- Preoperative desk telephone is usually busy. The Business Office cannot get through.
- The front desk does not know when patients are taken back for a preoperative visit. They often do not know that patients are waiting.
- Not enough registered nurses are available to see patients during preoperative visits.

The team acknowledged that the preoperative process was large and complex. To narrow the improvement effort, the team decided to try to improve the time that patients had to wait after they completed their paperwork and the nurse took them back for their preoperative interview.

The quality improvement director investigated how long patients should be expected to wait. As part of her investigation, she

- Asked patients, nurses, and business office staff what their perception of a delay was.
- Asked the business office to track how long it took patients to fill out their paperwork. Front desk staff determined that, on average, it took patients 15 to 20 minutes. Older patients or patients with disabilities (for example, cataracts) took longer.
- Interviewed local physician offices to see what they thought was a reasonable time for patients to wait to see a physician. She discovered that the community standard was between 15 and 30 minutes.

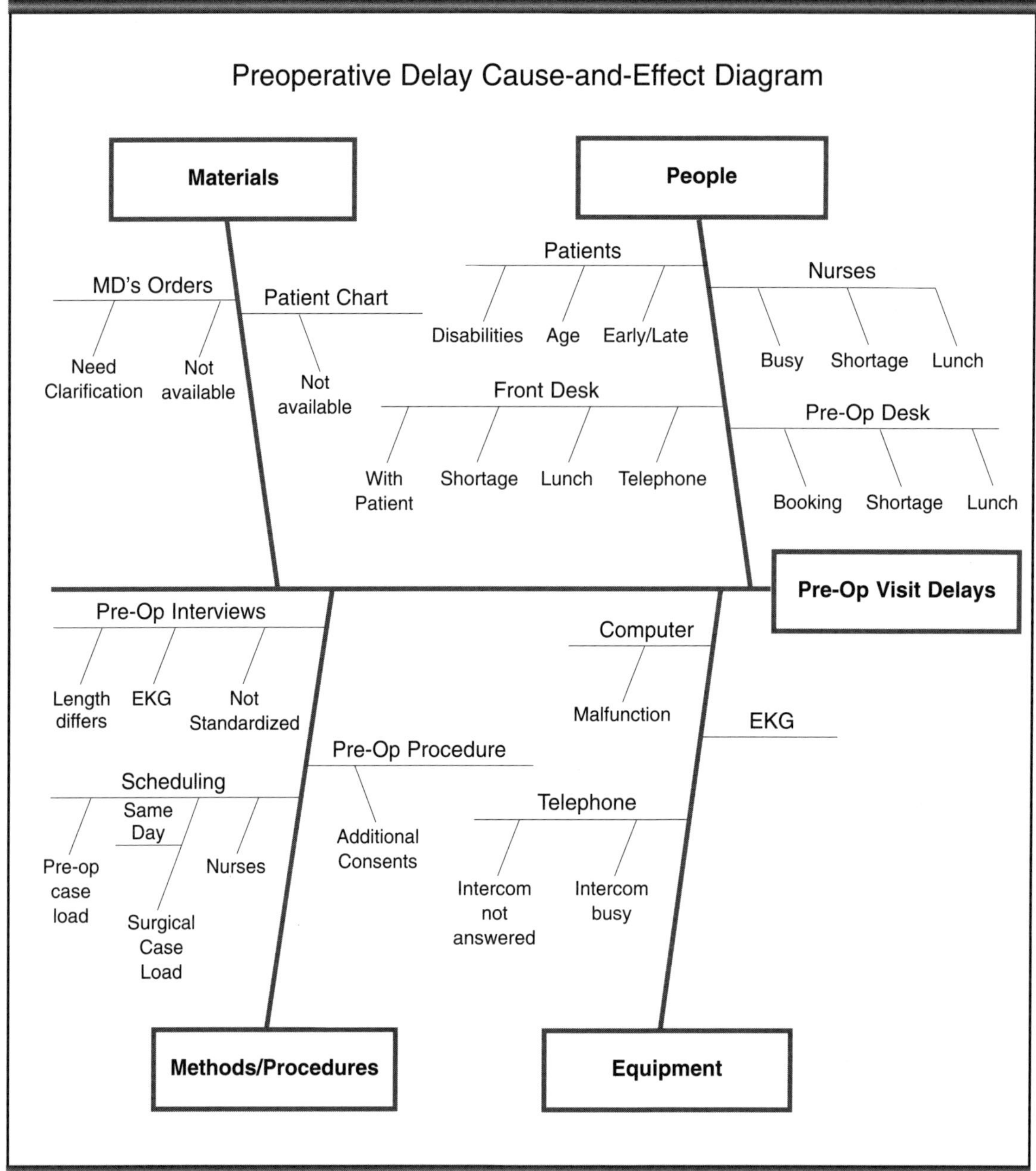

Figure 5-7. The team brainstormed sources of delays in the preop process and placed them in a cause-and-effect diagram.
Source: **Tallahassee Single Day Surgery Center, Tallahassee, FL. Used with permission.**

Based on this research, the team decided that preoperative patients should not have to wait any longer than 15 minutes to see a nurse after they completed their paperwork. In August and November 1993, staff collected data on how long preop patients waited. Data revealed that the surgery center was actually doing very well compared to the community standard. On average, patients only waited 8 minutes to see a nurse after completing their paperwork. Seventy-nine percent of the patients were seen within 15 minutes or less, and 92% of all patients were seen within 30 minutes.

Select the Process Improvement

Based on their data collection, managers realized that communication barriers between nursing and the business office were the main problem. To address this, team members brainstormed three possible solutions:

- Automate preoperative visits;
- Implement an electronic mail (e-mail) system that the business office and nursing can use to communicate patient arrivals; and
- Establish a process for exchanging paperwork between the two departments.

Because automating the preoperative process was unlikely at this time, the team decided to implement the last two solutions.

PDCA

The front desk and preoperative desk personnel were trained to use e-mail to communicate with each other regarding a patient's arrival. This eliminated finger pointing between the two departments. The two departments also established a way to exchange patients' paperwork. When nurses come out to the lobby to get a patient for their preoperative interview, they also picked up that patient's paperwork. This helped the front desk know which patients received a preoperative visit and which ones did not.

Results

After both these interventions were implemented, the team collected data on patient waiting times for two months (December 1993 and January 1994). A 5% improvement occurred in the amount of time patients had to wait to see a nurse after completing their paperwork (see Figure 5-8, page 148). The percentage of patients seen in 15 minutes or less increased from 79% to 84%.

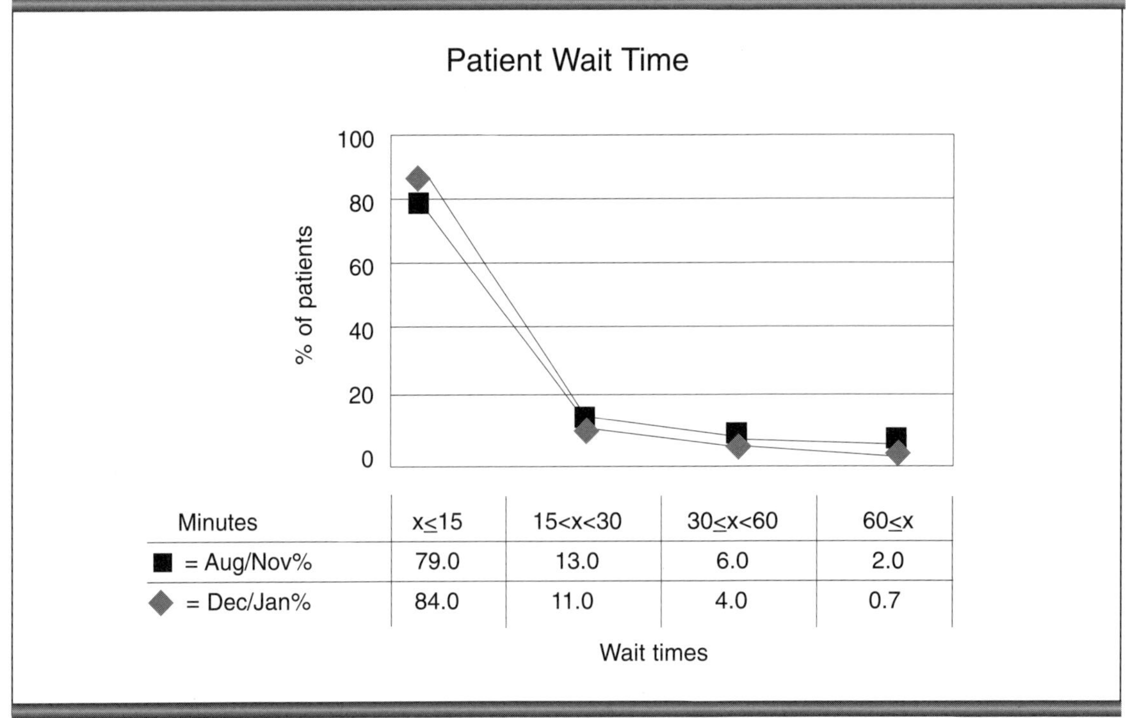

Minutes	x≤15	15<x<30	30≤x<60	60≤x
■ = Aug/Nov%	79.0	13.0	6.0	2.0
◆ = Dec/Jan%	84.0	11.0	4.0	0.7

Figure 5-8. After improvements were implemented to the preoperative process, patient wait times improved by 5%.
***Source:* Tallahasse Single Day Surgery Center, Tallahasee, FL. Used with permission.**

Equally important, communication between the two departments improved and the quality improvement director did not receive any written or verbal complaints from patients or staff regarding the process.

Staff became more sensitive to patient waiting times and realized that even occasional long wait times can increase a patient's anxiety, which affects his or her outcomes and satisfaction. Currently, nurses are trying to streamline and improve the preoperative interview portion of the process.

Example 5-3. Improving the Mammography Experience at a Radiology Center

Central Radiology Center, a hypothetical freestanding center in California, has 13 radiologists. The center's administrator, James Smith, notes that 15% of women are not showing up for their scheduled mammography appointments. James wants to decrease this appointment failure rate and increase the number of women who access the facility. To achieve these goals, he works with Susan Decker, administrative support, to explore how the center can reduce patient no-shows.

Example Highlights

Setting:
Central Radiology Center, Anycity, California

Performance Improvement Initiative:
Reduce patient no-shows while improving patient satisfaction.

Dimensions of Performance Addressed:
Effectiveness, efficiency, respect and caring.

Comments:
This example illustrates a two-pronged approach to performance improvement.

Identifying Solutions

James and Susan hold a focus group with 15 women who have just undergone the procedure. They discover that the radiology group could increase patient compliance with their scheduled appointments if they scheduled mammography appointments at more convenient times for the patients. They learn that the patients preferred not to come in on Saturday, as patients were often busy with weekend errands and activities. Susan tests various schedules for several months and identifies alternating weekday mornings and evenings as the best times for the patients.

James also wants to improve the patient's understanding of the procedure and make the experience less stressful. To this end, Laura Michaels, RN, develops written instructions for the patients that explain the nature of the mammography testing, what the patient can expect, and what preparation the patient must complete. The clinical staff then review, modify, and approve the educational materials. Susan also begins calling patients the day before their scheduled appointment to remind them of it and to see if they have any questions.

Measuring Improvement

To measure the success of these improvement interventions, James implements three performance measures:

- Appointment cancellations for mammography;
- No-show appointments for mammography; and
- A patient satisfaction questionnaire.

Within six months of implementing the changes, James finds that the canceled/no-show appointment rate dropped to 9% and, fewer women are unprepared or late for their appointments.

To track patient satisfaction, all patients are asked to fill out a card after their mammogram that asks one question: "Describe in two sentences or less your experiences today." These cards are dated so staff can identify problems by specific days. Feedback has been very positive. Patients describe the experience as "convenient," "professional," and "kind."

References

Assess for Success: Achieving Excellence with Joint Commission Standards and Baldrige Criteria. Oakbrook Terrace, IL: Joint Commission, 1997.

Bower KA: Developing and using critical paths. In: Lord JT (ed): *The Physician Leader's Guide.* Rockville, MD: Bader & Associates, Inc, pp 61–66, 1992.

Moore CH: *Quality Management in Health Care* 2/2 pp 13–26, Winter, 1994.

Weber DO: Clinical pathways stretch patient care but shrink costly lengths of stay at Anne Arundel Medical Center in Annapolis, Maryland. *Strategies for Healthcare Excellence.* pp 1–11, 1992.

Zander K: Critical pathways. In Melum MM, Sinioris MK (eds): *Total Quality Management: The Health Care Pioneers.* Chicago: American Hospital Publishing, Inc, pp 305–314, 1992.

CHAPTER 6: Examples

Chapter Highlights

This chapter presents two examples illustrating the entire performance improvement cycle–design, measure, assess, and improve.

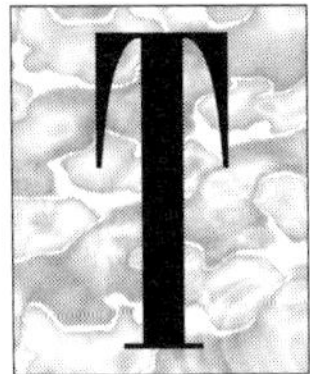

The examples in this chapter, as well as throughout this book, show that a variety of performance improvement approaches can be used and that a wide range of functions can be improved. The examples also illustrate the varying complexity of improvement activities. Equally important is the tenacity, teamwork, and creativity evident in these examples of performance improvement and the possibilities inherent in the Joint Commission's framework for improving performance. Finally, these examples demonstrate the value of a comprehensive, systematic approach to quality improvement.

Example Highlights

Setting:
Federal Correctional Institution (FCI) Terminal Island, Los Angeles/Long Beach Harbor, California

Performance Improvement Initiative:
Reduce patient waiting time to receive medical attention and increase patient and staff satisfaction.

Dimensions of Performance Addressed:
Availability, efficiency, timeliness.

Comments:
This example illustrates how an organization can dramatically improve a process by formalizing policies and procedures, and instituting some simple improvements.

Example 6-1. Improving the Sick Call System at a Correctional Facility

The Setting and Background

The Federal Correctional Institution (FCI), Terminal Island, is a medium-security federal prison located in the Los Angeles/Long Beach Harbor. It is also the Bureau of Prison's Western Region Medical Referral Center. Built in 1938, this facility houses 1,200 adult male inmates. Inmates range in age from 18 to 80 years old and most of the inmates are healthy. Approximately 200 inmates who have chronic illnesses and visit a physician or physician's assistant on a quarterly basis.

Inmate health care is provided by the health services unit. It is an ambulatory care clinic with a 13-bed short stay unit. The clinic and short stay unit are staffed around the clock. Inmates who are not enrolled in the chronic care clinic typically receive medical care via the sick call, same-day appointment system. In addition, inmates from other Bureau of Prison institutions are sent to Terminal Island for evaluation of medical problems.

The Problem

Prior to this study, inmates frequently voiced complaints concerning the amount of time it took to be seen for a medical problem. Health services staff also had difficulties seeing the large number of inmates who reported for sick call and finding time to complete appropriate documentation. In addition, patient follow-up was difficult due to misplaced or incomplete paperwork.

The institution's governing body asked the Committee of the Whole (COW), the health services' quality management group, to study the problem. After reviewing the issue, the COW assigned a CQI team to identify and implement solutions.

The Project Team

The multidisciplinary CQI team was created, which included members of Terminal Island's correctional staff, UNICOR (Prison Industries), and managers and counselors from several housing units, food service, and facility maintenance. Health services staff on the team included the Supervisory Physician's Assistant, Assistant Health Services Administrator, and the Quality Management Coordinator, who was also the team facilitator. The Associate Warden of Operations, who is a member of the governing body, sent a memo outlining the team's purpose to all departments within the institution. The team met monthly for approximately one hour.

Defining the Problem

Team members immediately decided that they needed to measure and document the extent of the problem. They asked a group of 10 physician's assistants to collect data and information that would help define the current sick call process.

The physician assistants reviewed sick call logs and outpatient records to determine the number of sick call patients seen and the severity of the patients' problems. The group also interviewed physicians to obtain their perspective. The group's findings included the following:

- The average number of inmates seen each day was 52;
- The average number of staff performing sick call was three; and
- A great deal of time was spent
  - retrieving medical records that were located in a different part of the building,
  - changing dressings throughout the day, and
  - handling walk-ins and call-ins who were frequently of a nonemergency nature.

Solidifying the Team

The team reviewed the physician assistants' report, and then conducted some brainstorming to produce additional ideas about the problem. The ideas were then grouped in terms of similarity and prioritized from the most to the least important cause of sick call problems. Some of these ideas included:

- Health services was not represented at the intermittent health care unit (IHC) during unit town hall meetings on Wednesdays. (The IHC is a housing unit that is physically modified to meet handicap regulations. Inmates are placed in the IHC for various reasons, such as being wheelchair bound or being an insulin-dependent diabetic.)
- The chronic care physician's assistant was not always available to see inmates in the IHC on a twice weekly basis.
- Psychology services were not available in the IHC.
- It was difficult to get appointments for food service and outside crew (gate pass) inmates.
- No additional staff could be added due to government cutbacks.

The team concluded that sick calls were currently handled in a haphazard fashion and decided to develop a formal procedure for how sick calls would be handled. They conducted some informal benchmarking to investigate and review how other institutions conducted sick call.

Team members interviewed staff at these institutions about how they handled sick call and requested copies of their sick call policies.

See page 96 for a discussion on benchmarking.

Interventions

One of the organizations interviewed, MCC San Diego, had achieved a dramatic 75% drop in the number of sick call appointments and inmates had expressed satisfaction with the system. Instead of developing a new sick call system from scratch, the team decided to examine what was working well at MCC San Diego and adapt the policies to fit their local resources and environment.

Team members kept in mind that inmates often try to maneuver within the system to avoid work details, seek drugs, and manipulate staff for their own purposes. For this reason, the team determined that the new sick call process had to incorporate the following factors:

- The system would have to be consistent.
- Inmate contact would need to be increased to promote their cooperation and decrease their perception that new rules meant less availability of health care.
- Patient satisfaction would have to be an ongoing activity. Written questionnaires were better suited for this environment. Statements made anonymously and in private tended to be a lot different from verbal responses, especially if an inmate felt he was being heard by other inmates.

Once completed, the new sick call procedure formalized the following:

- The day duty physician's assistant would triage patients starting at 0615 hours.
- Medical records personnel would bring charts of patients who are being triaged to the ambulatory care area.
- Sick call would start at 0800 hours. Slot appointments would be issued depending on the severity of the problem. Afternoons would be for patient follow-ups, procedures, hearing tests, and so forth.
- Unit officers and work supervisors would be required to call the duty physician assistant before sending any inmate to the ambulatory care unit.
- Walk-ins would not be permitted unless it was a life-threatening condition.
- Dressing changes would be done from 1200 to 1230 hours.
- Blood pressure checks would be performed by the Chronic Care Coordinator.

The team submitted the new sick call procedure to the COW and the governing body for their approval. Once it was approved, the team carried out the following to ensure that the new policy was implemented:

- The new policy was discussed at staff meetings and posted on staff bulletin boards.
- Other institution staff members were notified of the changes being made, their responsibilities, and the scheduled date of implementation. They were also invited to visit health services to observe and ask questions.
- Physician's assistants were given instruction on how to triage patients.
- The day-watch physicians assistants now reported to work at 0600 so they could work with the morning-watch physician's assistant to triage sick call patients.
- Health services staff were made available at food service during lunch to answer questions that any inmate might have.
- Lay-ins would not be issued during triage since inmates rarely kept the subsequent appointment. (A "lay-in" is a medical absence from an inmate work assignment for up to three days.) The inmates were assigned to their bunks except for eating and bathroom privileges.

Results and Outcomes

Six months later, a follow-up study revealed that the number of sick calls had dropped nearly 50% to an average of 27 per day (see Figure 6-1, page 158).

See page 103 for a discussion on histograms.

Concurrently, medical records reported that the time it took staff to transcribe results from laboratories and special studies into the charts had drastically improved from weeks to days.

The physician's assistants reported less stress and more job satisfaction, and unit managers and work supervisors reported that they heard fewer complaints from the inmates. Also, correctional staff were better able to account for the status and location of inmates, which is extremely important in a prison population.

Most important, however, is that patient satisfaction increased with reduced waiting time to be seen for a medical complaint. Custody and unit staff from all areas of the institution noted a dramatic difference. Inmates rarely complained about health services, and from 1994 to 1995, inmate suits against health services dropped 27%.

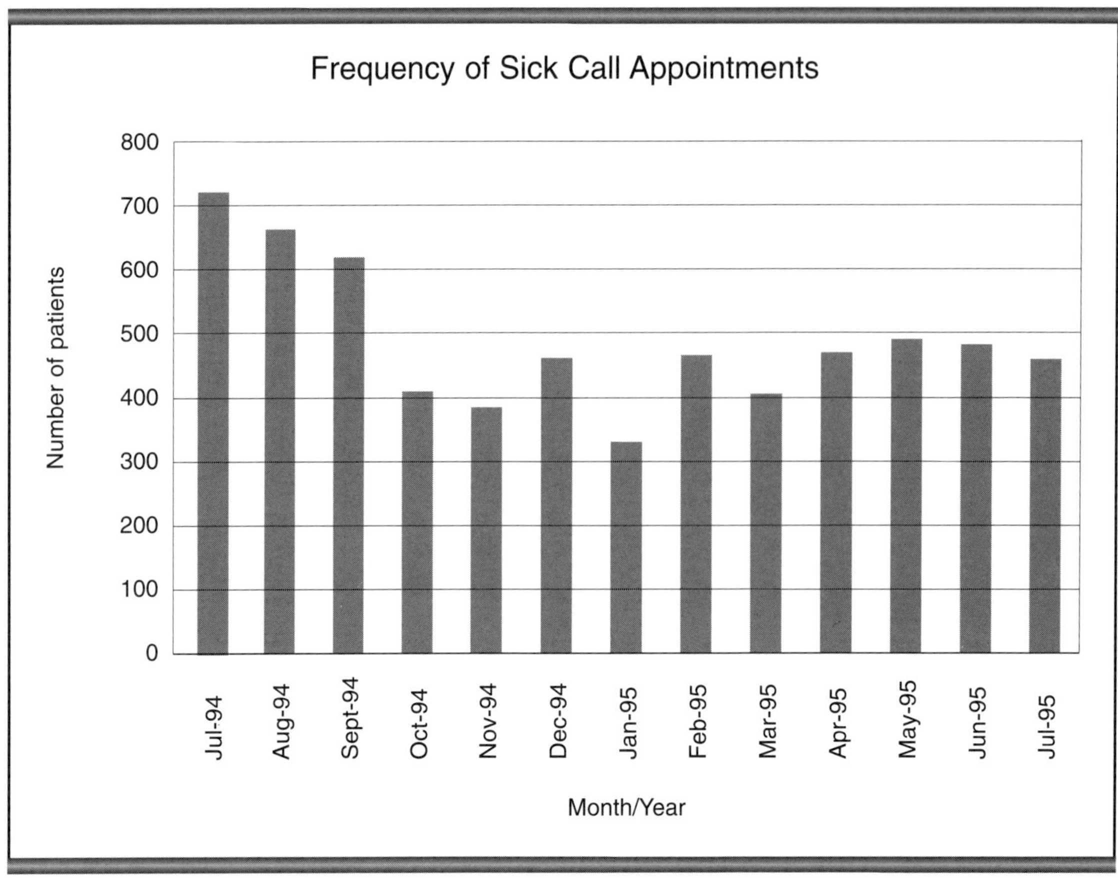

Figure 6-1. After implementing the new sick call process, the health services unit saw the number of sick calls drop significantly.
Source: **Federal Correctional Institution, Terminal Island, Los Angeles/Long Beach Harbor, CA. Used with permission.**

Example 6-2. Reorganization of the Walk-in Clinic at a Veterans Affairs Medical Center

The Setting and Background

The Jerry L. Pettis Memorial Veterans Affairs Medical Center (VAMC), Loma Linda, California, is a large, suburban medical center that offers comprehensive care to veterans and their families within a 200-mile radius. The ambulatory care center is a department within the medical center and saw 25,500 patients in 1995, which translated into 207,068 visits.

The VAMC has been involved in performance improvement activities since 1992, measuring various performance indicators and conducting improvement efforts on a regular basis. Staff typically follow the FOCUS-PDCA problem-solving approach.

See page 131 for a discussion of FOCUS-PDCA problem solving.

Example Highlights

Setting:
Jerry L. Pettis Memorial Veterans Affairs Medical Center (VAMC), Loma Linda, California

Performance Improvement Initiative:
Create a patient scheduling system that will reduce patient waiting times, reduce overtime costs, and increase patient and staff satisfaction.

Dimensions of Performance Addressed:
Appropriateness, availability, efficiency, timeliness.

Comments:
This example illustrates how a team uses benchmarking to create a scheduling system.

The Problem

Prior to March 1995, patients literally walked into the ambulatory care center's Walk-in Clinic without an appointment. Approximately 40 patients had scheduled appointments each day. Many additional patients came on their own; some were sent by other departments in the VAMC. In the past, the medical center used the Walk-in Clinic as the site of care for all patients without an assigned provider (that is, approximately 50% of VAMC patients did not have an assigned primary care physician in 1995).

Ambulatory care staff were frustrated by unstructured patient flow process. The patient load was continually increasing, averaging 83 to 96 patients per day. Due to fluctuation in the daily census, managers had difficulty ensuring that staffing levels matched the number of patients. This led to long hours for nurses, physicians, and others, as well as high overtime costs.

Patients were also dissatisfied with waiting times that averaged more than three hours and sometimes exceeded six hours. In addition, most patients thought the system was complicated and were frustrated with the poor morale and service among clinic staff.

In November 1994, ambulatory care department leaders decided to tackle this problem. After receiving approval from the VAMC's Performance Improvement

Committee, they assigned a project team to identify and implement appropriate improvements.

The Project Team

The eight-member project team included an interdisciplinary mix of nurses, clerical staff, supervisors, and physicians. Team members were selected from those staff that actually worked in the Walk-in Clinic as well as those who were administratively responsible for its function. Those team members not familiar with continuous quality improvement (CQI) went through formal training. The project team met for two months.

Defining the Problem

Team members began by discussing why everyone including patients, nurses, clerical staff, and physicians was frustrated with the current system in the Walk-in Clinic. Using the brainstorming tool, the team generated a list of important issues that made the system nonuser friendly:

- The number of patients who used the Walk-in Clinic varied from day to day;
- It was hard to adjust the staffing ratio since it was difficult to predict the number of patients;
- The total number of patients coming to the Walk-in Clinic was increasing;
- There were a limited number of staff available to care for patients in the Walk-in Clinic;
- Patients experienced long waiting times—up to six or eight hours;
- Extensive overtime for nursing, clerical, and pharmacy staff; and
- The lack of ability to quickly obtain the medical chart of walk-in patients.

Benchmarking

See page 96 for a discussion on benchmarking.

The team decided to find out how other ambulatory care clinics schedule patient appointments. Team members gathered benchmark information from several sources:

- An electronic on-line forum sponsored by the VA system. Like similar systems on the Internet, ambulatory care managers can share ideas with other managers in the VA system by sending e-mails back and forth. The problem of patient walk-in scheduling was a hot topic on the forum at this time, and the team was able to obtain several examples of how other systems handle the problem.
- District meetings for ambulatory care managers in the VA system. The ambulatory care managers brought back ideas on patient scheduling from their bi-monthly meetings with other VAMCs in southern California.
- Telephone conversations with local urgent care centers to learn how they handled patient scheduling.

Planning the Change

The team decided that some type of appointment scheduling system needed to be put in place and decided to change the name of the clinic from "Walk-in Clinic" to "Urgent Care Clinic." Team members felt that this name change would stress to patients and other VAMC providers that patients could no longer simply walk into the clinic.

The team elected to modify an urgent care system pioneered at the Memphis VAMC by Sarah Carter, MD. This system is based on two simple and related concepts: scheduled appointments and telephone triage. If the medical problem is minor, the clerk makes an appointment for the patient to see a physician. The clerk transfers all other calls to a triage nurse who follows pre-established protocols to determine the urgency of the patient's problem and if they need an appointment. The nurse also provides patients with self-care instructions when applicable.

Team members determined what needed to be done to adapt a similar system in their Urgent Care Clinic. This included:

- Recruiting and training triage nurses. Two nurses from the medical center's ICU were recruited and trained to operate as triage nurses.
- Develop triage protocols. Ambulatory care physicians and the triage nurses developed triage protocols for 27 different patient scenarios. These protocols were symptom-based guidelines that help the triage nurse determine the appropriate course of care for a patient (see Figure 6-2, page 162, for an example of a headache protocol).
- Prepare ambulatory care staff for new system. Team members held several role-playing sessions with clinic clerks and nurses to prepare them

Triage Protocols for Registered Nurses

The Protocols are designed to classify the patient's problem (chief complaint) into five categories as follows:

Emergent patient problems: The patient should be directed to call 911 or report to the Emergency Room.

Urgent: The patient should be instructed to report for a same-day appointment. This appointment should be arranged immediately.

Non-urgent: The patient should be seen within 2–5 days in the assigned module, clinic, or urgent care.

Routine: The patient should be seen within 2 weeks in the assigned module, clinic, or urgent care.

Patient Education: The reported problem does not warrant medical evaluation but the patient should be evaluated for new patient or follow-up evaluation.

The nurse cannot see or touch the patient during telephone interview and must rely on information received through directed questioning, communicated caring, and an understanding that neither the patient nor the significant other have medical knowledge. The triage nurse may not have access to the patient's medical record during the interview. Therefore, the nurse must gather information in the most accurate manner possible to guarantee safe disposition of the problem. The Protocol format has an X for the action of reported symptoms.

Problem/Chief Complaint/Symptom	911/ER	Same-Day Consult MD	2–5 Days	2 Weeks	Patient Education
HEADACHE					X
Confused or not acting normal —sudden onset	X				
Difficulty with speaking or slurred speech	X				
Unsteady walking or weakness	X				
Difficult to arouse	X				
Blurred or double vision	X				
Vomiting—more than three times	X				
Change in mental status (person, place, time, date)	X				
Pupils unequal (determined by S/O)	X				
Associated with fever > 101, stiff neck, delirium	X				
New Pain—severe or sudden onset—region of pain		X			
No relief or worse after home treatment		X			

Figure 6-2. As part of their new urgent care system, the VAMC clinic developed symptom-based triage protocols to help triage nurses determine the appropriate course of care for a patient. The above protocol focuses on headaches.
Source: **Jerry L. Pettis Memorial Veterans Affairs Medical Center, Loma Linda, CA. Used with permission.**

Figure 6-2 continued.

Triage Protocols for Registered Nurses–continued

Problem/Chief Complaint/Symptom	911/ER	Same-Day Consult MD	2–5 Days	2 Weeks	Patient Education
Migraine—recurring		X			
Proceeded by visual changes—N/V—Aura			X		
Pain on one side of head—near eye brow			X		
Throbbing, dull, constant, mild—generalized			X		
Symptoms mild			X		
History of allergies or sinusitis				X	
Current medications		X			

PATIENT EDUCATION:

Severe Headache: Urge patient to seek medical care and *not to drive.*

Migraine Headache: Rest in dark quiet room. Place cool compresses to head. Massage hollows at base of skull.

***Call back if headache lasts longer than 12 hours, headache becomes worse, new symptoms develop.**

Sinus Headache: Take prescribed antihistamines, Tylenol, or Motrin.

for how to handle various patient scenarios under the new appointment system. For example, staff acted out what should happen when a patient walks into the clinic without an appointment or when a patient with back pain calls.

- Communicating changes to patients. This included reviewing the change in process with local Veteran's Service Organizations, placing descriptive posters in prominent places in the facility, and sending letters to all patients explaining the change.
- Obtaining the buy-in of all VAMC staff. Prior to initiating the changes in the system, the team sent letters to all service chiefs and physicians outlining the system overhaul and discussed the changes at facilitywide employee forums.

Initiating the New Process

On March 15, 1995, the team initiated the telephone triage and scheduled appointment systems in the newly named Urgent Care Clinic. Patients and staff willingly accepted the change with minimal complaints.

Results

Over the first 11 months of the clinic's reorganization, the clinic has seen significant benefits:

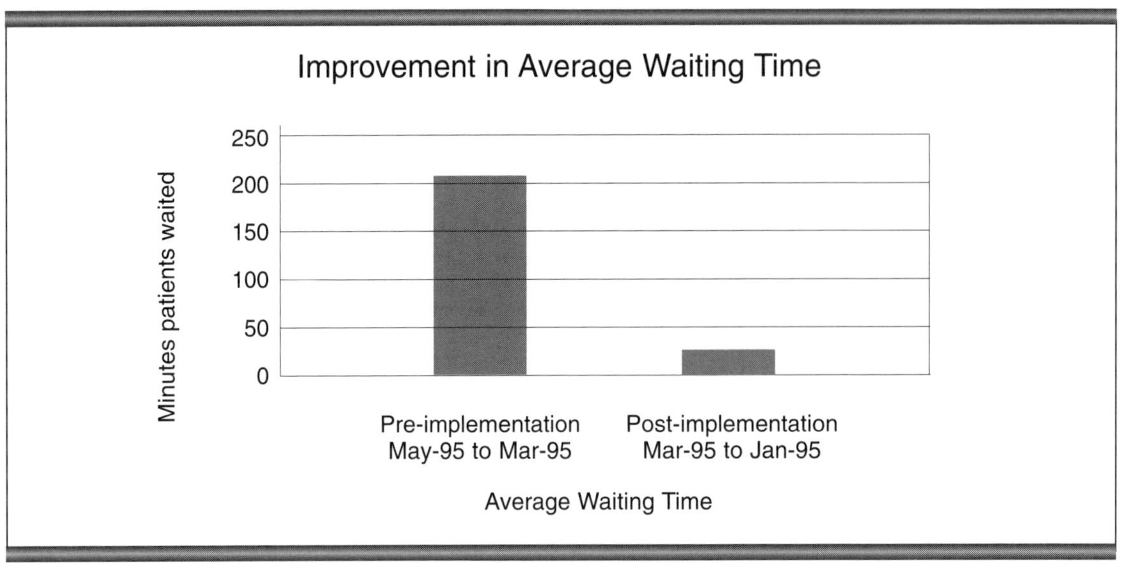

Figure 6-3. Waiting times improved dramatically in the urgent care clinic. Most patients are now seen within 30 minutes of their scheduled appointment.
Source: **Jerry L. Pettis Memorial Veterans Affairs Medical Center, Loma Linda, CA. Used with permission.**

- Decreased waiting time. Most patients are seen within 30 minutes of their scheduled appointment (see Figure 6-3, above).

See page 103 for a discussion on histograms.

- Decrease in urgent care census. The number of patients seen has fallen from an average of 87 per day (with a high of 120) to an average of 76 per day (with a high of 90) (see Figure 6-4, page 165).
- Minimal overtime for nurses, clerks, pharmacy personnel, and physicians.
- Increased patient satisfaction.

Staff continue to monitor the process to ensure that the clinic maintains this improved level of service. They track three performance measures on a monthly basis: the number of patients seen, the number of people who continue to walk into the clinic, and the number of patient complaints.

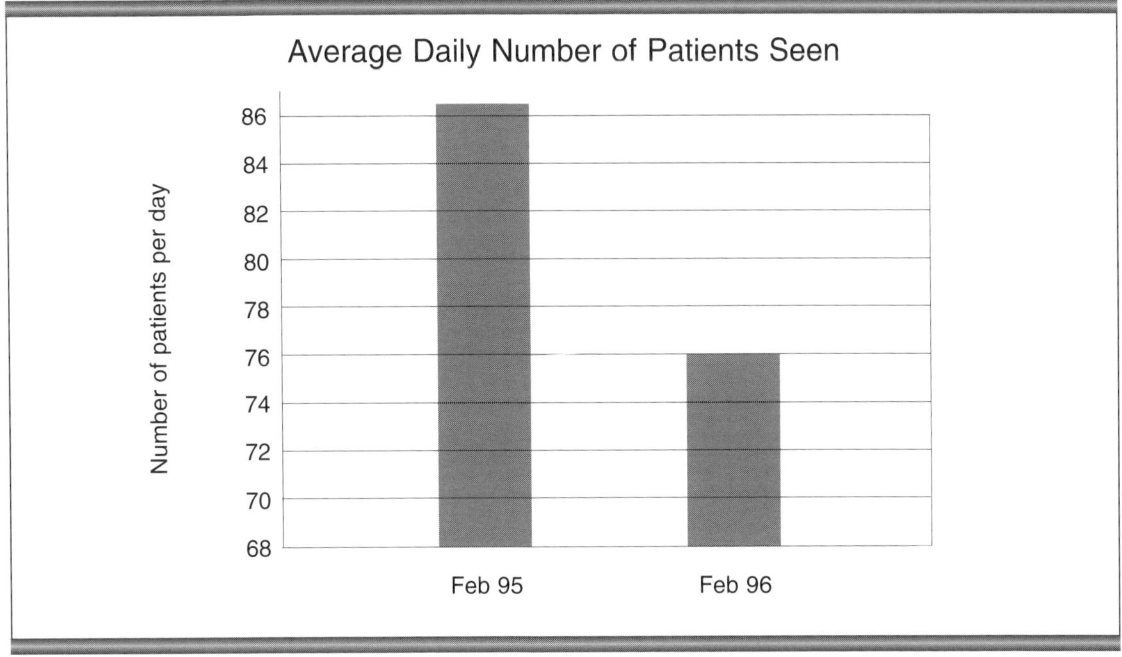

Figure 6-4. The number of patients seen has fallen from an average of 87 per day to an average of 76 per day.
Source: **Jerry L. Pettis Memorial Veterans Affairs Medical Center, Loma Linda, CA. Used with permission.**

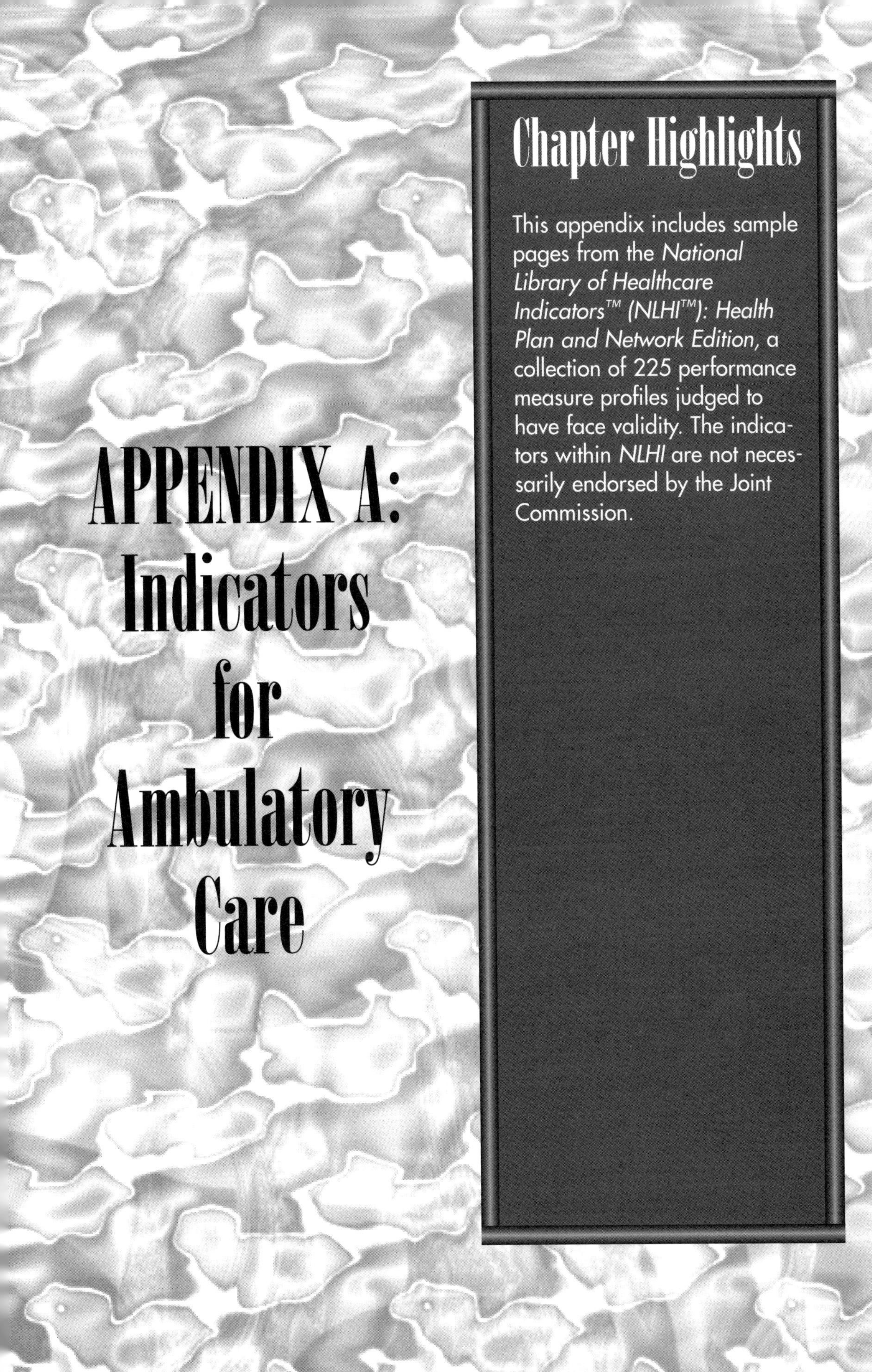

APPENDIX A: Indicators for Ambulatory Care

Chapter Highlights

This appendix includes sample pages from the *National Library of Healthcare Indicators™ (NLHI™): Health Plan and Network Edition,* a collection of 225 performance measure profiles judged to have face validity. The indicators within *NLHI* are not necessarily endorsed by the Joint Commission.

Clinical Performance
Health Status

Arthritis

PERFORMANCE MEASURE PROFILE

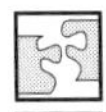 *Appropriateness*

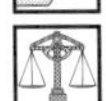 *Efficacy*

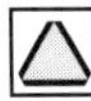 *Prevention/Early Detection*

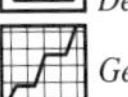 *General Health*

PERFORMANCE MEASURE
Monitoring osteoarthritis.

FOCUS OF MEASURE
Routine monitoring of chronic conditions.

RATIONALE
Osteoarthritis is a chronic disease that requires continuing evaluation.

TYPE OF MEASURE
Process

NUMERATOR STATEMENT
Patients 65 years of age or older with osteoarthritis who are appropriately monitored.

Numerator Description
Data Element(s): Presence of monitoring item

Corresponding Data Source(s): Medical record

Included Populations: Appropriate annual monitoring includes control of symptoms documentation, examination of joints most affected, weight measurement, and medication side effects.

Excluded Populations: None

DENOMINATOR STATEMENT
Patients 65 years of age or older with osteoarthritis.

Denominator Description
Data Element(s):
A. Date of birth
B. Diagnosis of osteoarthritis

Corresponding Data Source(s):
A. Claims data
B. Medical record

Included Populations: Patients with osteoarthritis

Excluded Populations: Patients younger than 65 years of age

DOMAINS OF PERFORMANCE

Domain	
Appropriateness	Yes
Availability	No
Continuity	No
Effectiveness	No
Efficacy	Yes
Efficiency	No
Prevention/Early Detection	Yes
Respect and Caring	No
Safety	No
Timeliness	No

DELIVERY SETTINGS	Initial Settings	Applicable Settings
Health Care Network/Plan	✓	✓
Hospital		
Practitioner Office	✓	✓
Ambulatory Care Clinic	✓	✓
Behavioral Health		
Home Care		
Nursing Home		
Subacute Care Setting		
Rehabilitation Setting		
Hospice		
Clinical Laboratory		

TESTING

Testing	
Reliability	Yes
Validity	Yes
Relevance	Yes
Discriminatory Capability	Yes
Data Collection Effort	Yes
Denominator Verification	No

Continued on following page

0124-00292

Continued from previous page

STRATIFICATION
Yes

RISK ADJUSTMENT
Yes

CURRENT DEVELOPMENT STATUS
Pilot testing is complete but measure is not yet implemented.

ADDITIONAL INFORMATION
Each monitor (for example, control of symptoms documentation) is a separate indicator rate.

SUBMITTING ORGANIZATION
Harvard School of Public Health
Profile confirmed March 1996

ORIGINAL PERFORMANCE MEASURE SOURCE/DEVELOPER
A Project to Develop and Evaluate Methods to Promote Ambulatory Care Quality (DEMPAQ)

PERFORMANCE MEASURE
Prevention—mammogram.

FOCUS OF MEASURE
Appropriate provision of preventive services on a routine basis.

RATIONALE
The effectiveness of clinical examination of the breast combined with mammography has been shown by several studies.

TYPE OF MEASURE
Process

NUMERATOR STATEMENT
Number of women 65-75 years old who have a mammogram done once in a two-year period.

Numerator Description
Data Element(s): Mammogram present

Corresponding Data Source(s): Medical record

Included Populations: Not applicable

Excluded Populations: None

DENOMINATOR STATEMENT
Number of women 65-75 years old.

Denominator Description
Data Element(s):

A. Date of birth
B. Gender

Corresponding Data Source(s):

A-B. Medical record; administrative data

Included Populations: Not applicable

Excluded Populations: Male patients; female patients younger than 65 years or older than 75 years

DOMAINS OF PERFORMANCE
Appropriateness . . . . Yes
Availability . . . . Yes
Continuity . . . . No
Effectiveness . . . . No
Efficacy . . . . No
Efficiency . . . . No
Prevention/Early Detection . . . . Yes
Respect and Caring . . . . No
Safety . . . . No
Timeliness . . . . No

DELIVERY SETTINGS	Initial Settings	Applicable Settings
Health Care Network/Plan	✓	✓
Hospital		
Practitioner Office		
Ambulatory Care Clinic	✓	✓
Behavioral Health		
Home Care		
Nursing Home		
Subacute Care Setting		
Rehabilitation Setting		
Hospice		
Clinical Laboratory		

TESTING
Reliability . . . . Yes
Validity . . . . Yes
Relevance . . . . Yes
Discriminatory Capability . . . . Yes
Data Collection Effort . . . . Yes
Denominator Verification . . . . No

STRATIFICATION
Yes

RISK ADJUSTMENT
Yes

CURRENT DEVELOPMENT STATUS
Pilot testing is complete but measure is not yet implemented.

ADDITIONAL INFORMATION
Not applicable

SUBMITTING ORGANIZATION
Harvard School of Public Health
Profile confirmed March 1996

ORIGINAL PERFORMANCE MEASURE SOURCE/DEVELOPER
A Project to Develop and Evaluate Methods to Promote Ambulatory Care Quality (DEMPAQ)

Clinical Performance
Health Status

Breast Cancer
Health Maintenance—Adult

PERFORMANCE MEASURE PROFILE

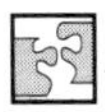
Appropriateness

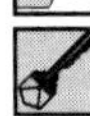
Availability

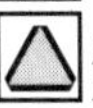
Prevention/Early Detection

General Health

0124-00300

Clinical Performance

Depression

PERFORMANCE MEASURE PROFILE

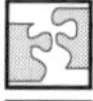 *Appropriateness*

 *Continuity*

 *Prevention/Early Detection*

 *Respect and Caring*

 *Safety*

 *Timeliness*

PERFORMANCE MEASURE

Outpatients diagnosed with depressive disorders without documented follow-up or a referral to a mental health care setting.

FOCUS OF MEASURE

Ongoing assessment and/or appropriate referral of patients with a depressive disorder in a primary care setting.

RATIONALE

Depression in a primary care setting is a highly treatable illness. With adequate doses of antidepressants, a significant improvement in depressive symptoms is commonly seen in 75% of patients in 4-8 weeks. However, recent studies conducted in HMOs found that 30-40% of patients who had been started on antidepressants dropped out of treatment within the first 30 days. This may have been related to several factors, one of which is a lack of close follow-up by the clinicians.

Regardless of the type of treatment a patient and practitioner select, frequent follow-up is vital during the initial stages of therapy. The depression's clinical course should be monitored until symptom relief becomes evident. This can be accomplished through regularly scheduled office visits or telephone contact. When a patient's symptoms do not improve or worsen, a psychiatric consultation should be considered. Through good follow-up and provision of appropriate treatment, perhaps a significant portion of those 30-40% who drop out of treatment can be helped, having a significant impact on the quality of life, work productivity, and health care dollars spent.

TYPE OF MEASURE

Process

NUMERATOR STATEMENT

Outpatients with a diagnosis of a depressive disorder in a primary care setting without documented follow-up for the diagnosis at that site or an appropriate referral to a mental health care setting for management of the depressive disorder.

Numerator Description

Data Element(s):

A. Documentation of continued assessment of depressed condition

B. Referral to mental health care setting/practitioner

Corresponding Data Source(s):

A-B. Measure not developed to the point of determining data sources

Included Populations: Outpatients without documented follow-up for the diagnosis at that site or an appropriate referral to a mental health care setting for managment of the depressive disorder

Excluded Populations: None

DENOMINATOR STATEMENT

Outpatients with a diagnosis of a depressive disorder in the primary care setting.

Denominator Description

Data Element(s): Diagnosis codes

Corresponding Data Source(s): Medical records

Included Populations: Outpatients with a diagnosis of a depressive disorder; primary care setting; code table available upon request from submitting organization

Excluded Populations: Inpatients

DOMAINS OF PERFORMANCE

Domain	
Appropriateness	Yes
Availability	No
Continuity	Yes
Effectiveness	No
Efficacy	No
Efficiency	No
Prevention/Early Detection	Yes
Respect and Caring	Yes
Safety	Yes
Timeliness	Yes

Continued on following page

DELIVERY SETTINGS

	Initial Settings	Applicable Settings
Health Care Network/Plan		✓
Hospital		
Practitioner Office		✓
Ambulatory Care Clinic		✓
Behavioral Health		✓
Home Care		
Nursing Home		
Subacute Care Setting		
Rehabilitation Setting		
Hospice		
Clinical Laboratory		

TESTING

Reliability . . . . No
Validity . . . . No
Relevance . . . . Yes
Discriminatory Capability. . . . . No
Data Collection Effort . . . . No
Denominator Verification . . . . No

STRATIFICATION

No

RISK ADJUSTMENT

No

CURRENT DEVELOPMENT STATUS

Measure defined but not yet pilot tested.

ADDITIONAL INFORMATION

Not applicable

SUBMITTING ORGANIZATION

Joint Commission on Accreditation of Healthcare Organizations (Joint Commission), Department of Research and Evaluation
Profile confirmed March 1996

ORIGINAL PERFORMANCE MEASURE SOURCE/DEVELOPER

Joint Commission

Clinical Performance

Depression

Continued from previous page

PERFORMANCE MEASURE

Appropriate response to an abnormal blood glucose test.

FOCUS OF MEASURE

Appropriate follow-up of abnormal test results (responding to information about the patient).

RATIONALE

Hypoglycemia in a nondiabetic may be caused by an organic problem which requires further workup and diagnosis. National Diabetes Data Group and World Health Organization standards require a repeat finding of abnormal plasma glucose levels before making a diagnosis of diabetes. If the patient is diabetic, control of blood glucose level prevents or delays many of the complications associated with diabetes.

TYPE OF MEASURE

Process

NUMERATOR STATEMENT

All patients 65 years of age or older who received an appropriate treatment response for an abnormal blood glucose level (fasting or random).

NUMERATOR DESCRIPTION

Data Element(s): Presence of appropriate treatment

Corresponding Data Source(s): Medical record

Included Populations: Not applicable

Excluded Populations: None

DENOMINATOR STATEMENT

All patients 65 years of age or older with a blood sugar less than 50 mg/dL or greater than 140 mg/dL (fasting not known to be diabetic), greater than 170 mg/dL (fasting, known to be diabetic), or greater than 250 mg/dL (random).

Denominator Description

Data Element(s):

A. Date of birth

B. Abnormal blood glucose test results

Corresponding Data Source(s):

A. Claims data

B. Medical records

Included Populations: Not applicable

Excluded Populations: Patients younger than 65 years of age

DOMAINS OF PERFORMANCE

Appropriateness .... Yes
Availability .... No
Continuity .... No
Effectiveness .... Yes
Efficacy .... No
Efficiency .... Yes
Prevention/Early Detection .... Yes
Respect and Caring .... No
Safety .... No
Timeliness .... Yes

DELIVERY SETTINGS

	Initial Settings	Applicable Settings
Health Care Network/Plan	✓	✓
Hospital		
Practitioner Office	✓	✓
Ambulatory Care Clinic	✓	✓
Behavioral Health		
Home Care		
Nursing Home		
Subacute Care Setting		
Rehabilitation Setting		
Hospice		
Clinical Laboratory		

TESTING

Reliability .... Yes
Validity .... Yes
Relevance .... Yes
Discriminatory Capability .... Yes
Data Collection Effort .... Yes
Denominator Verification .... No

Continued on following page

Clinical Performance

Diabetes

PERFORMANCE MEASURE PROFILE

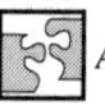 *Appropriateness*

 *Effectiveness*

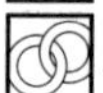 *Efficiency*

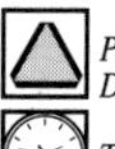 *Prevention/Early Detection*

Timeliness

0124-00317

Clinical Performance

Diabetes

Continued from previous page

STRATIFICATION

Yes

RISK ADJUSTMENT

Yes

CURRENT DEVELOPMENT STATUS

Pilot testing is complete but measure is not yet implemented.

ADDITIONAL INFORMATION

Not applicable

SUBMITTING ORGANIZATION

Harvard School of Public Health
Profile confirmed March 1996

ORIGINAL PERFORMANCE MEASURE SOURCE/DEVELOPER

A Project to Develop and Evaluate Methods to Promote Ambulatory Care Quality (DEMPAQ)

PERFORMANCE MEASURE

Member office visits to a primary care physician for management of hypertension, congestive heart failure, and diabetes mellitus.

FOCUS OF MEASURE

Access to care.

RATIONALE

Preventive and optimal management in chronic illnesses necessitates an office visit where that condition can be adequately monitored. Patients with a chronic disease should be seen in the physician office at least once per year for any change in condition, function, physical examination findings, medication regimen, and monitoring of key parameters.

TYPE OF MEASURE

Process

NUMERATOR STATEMENT

Number of members with the confirmed diagnosis of hypertension, congestive heart failure, or diabetes mellitus having at least one office visit to primary care physician during the monitored year for the primary purpose of management of that particular disease state.

Numerator Description

Data Element(s):

A. Diagnosis of hypertension
B. Diagnosis of congestive heart failure
C. Diagnosis of diabetes mellitus
D. Office visit

Corresponding Data Source(s):

A. Claims and encounter data: ICD-9-CM diagnosis codes 401.0 to 405.9; pharmacy database PTC/NDC code = 24:04
B. Claims and encounter data: ICD-9-CM diagnosis codes 428.0 to 428.9; pharmacy database PTC/NDC code = 24:04
C. Claims and encounter data: ICD-9-CM diagnosis codes 250.0 to 250.9; pharmacy database PTC/NDC code = 68:20.08 and 68:20.20
D. Claims and encounter data: CPT-4 = 99056; 99058; 99201 to 99205; 99211 to 99215; 99241 to 99245; 99271 to 99275; 99381 to 99387; 99391 to 99397; 99401 to 99404; 99411 to 99412; 99420; 99429 with ICD-9-CM diagnosis codes: 401.0 to 405.9; 642.0 to 642.3, 428.0 to 428.9, or 250.0 to 250.9

Included Populations: Not applicable

Excluded Populations: None

DENOMINATOR STATEMENT

Number of members (continuously enrolled for at least one year) with a confirmed diagnosis of hypertension, congestive heart failure, or diabetes mellitus.

Denominator Description

Data Element(s):

A. Enrolled throughout the monitored year
B. Diagnosis of hypertension
C. Diagnosis of congestive heart failure
D. Diagnosis of diabetes mellitus

Corresponding Data Source(s):

A. Enrollment data base
B. Claims and encounter data: ICD-9-CM diagnosis codes 401.0 to 405.9; pharmacy database PTC/NDC code = 24:04
C. Claims and encounter data: ICD-9-CM diagnosis codes 428.0 to 428.9; pharmacy database PTC/NDC code = 24:04
D. Claims and encounter data: ICD-9-CM diagnosis codes 250.0 to 250.9; pharmacy database PTC/NDC code = 68:20.08 and 68:20.20

Included Populations: All age groups, all patients who have one or more of the following three diagnoses: hypertension, congestive heart failure, diabetes mellitus. Diagnoses are confirmed by both appropriate ICD-9-CM diagnosis codes and appropriate drug usage.

Excluded Populations: None

DOMAINS OF PERFORMANCE

Domain	
Appropriateness	No
Availability	Yes
Continuity	No
Effectiveness	No
Efficacy	No
Efficiency	No
Prevention/Early Detection	Yes
Respect and Caring	No
Safety	No
Timeliness	Yes

Continued on following page

Clinical Performance
Health Status

Diabetes
Heart Disease
High Blood Pressure

PERFORMANCE MEASURE PROFILE

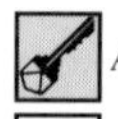
Availability

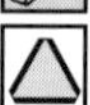
Prevention/Early Detection

Timeliness

General Health

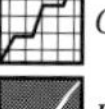
Reported Health Transition

Clinical Performance
Health Status

Diabetes
Heart Disease
High Blood Pressure

Continued from previous page

DELIVERY SETTINGS	Initial Settings	Applicable Settings
Health Care Network/Plan		✓
Hospital		
Practitioner Office	✓	✓
Ambulatory Care Clinic		
Behavioral Health		
Home Care		
Nursing Home		
Subacute Care Setting		
Rehabilitation Setting		
Hospice		
Clinical Laboratory		

TESTING

Reliability . . . . Yes
Validity . . . . Yes
Relevance . . . . No
Discriminatory Capability . . . . Yes
Data Collection Effort . . . . Yes
Denominator Verification . . . . No

STRATIFICATION

Yes

RISK ADJUSTMENT

No

CURRENT DEVELOPMENT STATUS

Measure was pilot tested and implemented.

ADDITIONAL INFORMATION

Not applicable

SUBMITTING ORGANIZATION

Humana, Inc

Profile confirmed February 1996

ORIGINAL PERFORMANCE MEASURE SOURCE/DEVELOPER

Humana, Inc

PERFORMANCE MEASURE

Appropriate response to an abnormal electrocardiogram (ECG) test.

FOCUS OF MEASURE

Appropriate follow up of abnormal test results (responding to information about the patient).

RATIONALE

Numerous drugs may affect cardiac rhythm and serum potassium balance. Before treating the arrhythmia with drugs the possible cause of the arrhythmia should be explored, especially thyroid dysfunction, congestive heart failure, electrolyte disturbance, pulmonary disease, or medications. A proper balance of serum potassium and calcium is necessary for normal cardiac muscle functioning, therefore, serum potassium and calcium levels should be evaluated.

TYPE OF MEASURE

Process

NUMERATOR STATEMENT

All patients 65 years of age or older who received an appropriate treatment response for an ECG test.

Numerator Description

Data Element(s): Presence of appropriate treatment

Corresponding Data Source(s): Medical record

Included Populations: Not applicable

Excluded Populations: None

DENOMINATOR STATEMENT

All patients with new onset rhythm disturbances other than sinus tachycardia or atrial fibrillation, stable bradycardia or stable trigeminy/quadrageminy, or patients with new atrial fibrillation or new metabolic changes on ECG.

Denominator Description

Data Element(s):

A. Date of birth
B. Abnormal ECG test results

Corresponding Data Source(s):

A. Claims data
B. Medical record

Included Populations: Not applicable

Excluded Populations: Patients younger than 65 years of age

DOMAINS OF PERFORMANCE

Appropriateness .... Yes
Availability .... No
Continuity .... No
Effectiveness .... Yes
Efficacy .... No
Efficiency .... Yes
Prevention/Early Detection .... Yes
Respect and Caring .... No
Safety .... No
Timeliness .... Yes

DELIVERY SETTINGS

	Initial Settings	Applicable Settings
Health Care Network/Plan	✓	✓
Hospital		
Practitioner Office	✓	✓
Ambulatory Care Clinic	✓	✓
Behavioral Health		
Home Care		
Nursing Home		
Subacute Care Setting		
Rehabilitation Setting		
Hospice		
Clinical Laboratory		

TESTING

Reliability .... Yes
Validity .... Yes
Relevance .... Yes
Discriminatory Capability .... Yes
Data Collection Effort .... Yes
Denominator Verification .... No

Continued on following page

Clinical Performance

Heart Disease

PERFORMANCE MEASURE PROFILE

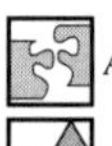
Appropriateness

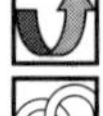
Effectiveness

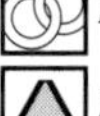
Efficiency

Prevention/Early Detection

Timeliness

0124-00324

Clinical Performance

Heart Disease

Continued from previous page

STRATIFICATION
Yes

RISK ADJUSTMENT
Yes

CURRENT DEVELOPMENT STATUS
Pilot testing is complete but measure is not yet implemented.

ADDITIONAL INFORMATION
Not applicable

SUBMITTING ORGANIZATION
Harvard School of Public Health
Profile confirmed March 1996

ORIGINAL PERFORMANCE MEASURE SOURCE/DEVELOPER
A Project to Develop and Evaluate Methods to Promote Ambulatory Care Quality (DEMPAQ)

Clinical Performance

Medication

PERFORMANCE MEASURE PROFILE

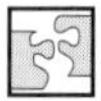 *Appropriateness*

 *Availability*

 *Continuity*

 *Effectiveness*

 *Efficacy*

 *Efficiency*

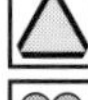 *Prevention/Early Detection*

 *Respect and Caring*

 *Safety*

 *Timeliness*

PERFORMANCE MEASURE

Selected surgical procedures for which prophylactic intravenous antibiotics were received: timing of prophylactic antibiotic administration.

FOCUS OF MEASURE

Timing of prophylactic intravenous antibiotic administration for selected surgical procedures.

RATIONALE

An essential principle of antibiotic prophylaxis is the achievement of adequate antibiotic serum and tissue concentrations prior to the surgical incision and throughout the procedure. Studies that have evaluated these practices commonly identify delays in timing of antibiotic administration in relation to surgery. The period immediately prior to surgical incision is considered the optimum time for administration of prophylactic antibiotics to reduce the risk for surgery-related infection.

TYPE OF MEASURE

Process

OTHER STATEMENT

Selected inpatient and outpatient surgical procedures for which prophylactic intravenous antibiotics were received: timing of prophylactic antibiotic administration.

Other Description

Data Element(s):

A. ICD-9-CM procedure codes
B. Procedure dates
C. Patient received antibiotic
D. Prophylactic antibiotic administration date
E. Prophylactic antibiotic administration time
F. Surgical incision time

Corresponding Data Source(s):

A-F. Medical record; billing data; UB-92

Included Populations: All inpatients, outpatients, and emergency department patients undergoing a selected surgical procedure from among any of 17 selected surgical procedure groups for which prophylactic intravenous antibiotics were received, reported by time of antibiotic administration prior to or after surgical incision by surgical procedure group. Selected surgical procedures are identified by the presence of a related ICD-9-CM procedure code. Each health care organization needs to determine its population of interest by choosing one or more of the 17 surgical procedure groups. Selected surgical groups and related ICD-9-CM procedure code tables are available upon request from the submitting organization.

Excluded Populations: None

DOMAINS OF PERFORMANCE

Domain	
Appropriateness	Yes
Availability	Yes
Continuity	Yes
Effectiveness	Yes
Efficacy	Yes
Efficiency	Yes
Prevention/Early Detection	Yes
Respect and Caring	Yes
Safety	Yes
Timeliness	Yes

DELIVERY SETTINGS	Initial Settings	Applicable Settings
Health Care Network/Plan		✓
Hospital	✓	✓
Practitioner Office		
Ambulatory Care Clinic		✓
Behavioral Health		
Home Care		
Nursing Home		
Subacute Care Setting		
Rehabilitation Setting		
Hospice		
Clinical Laboratory		

Continued on following page

0100-00033

Clinical Performance

Medication

Continued from previous page

TESTING

Reliability . . . . Yes
Validity . . . . Yes
Relevance . . . . Yes
Discriminatory Capability . . . . Yes
Data Collection Effort . . . . Yes
Denominator Verification . . . . No

STRATIFICATION

No

RISK ADJUSTMENT

No

CURRENT DEVELOPMENT STATUS

Measure was pilot tested and implemented.

ADDITIONAL INFORMATION

Not applicable

SUBMITTING ORGANIZATION

Joint Commission on Accreditation of Healthcare Organizations (Joint Commission), Indicator Measurement System (IMSystem®)
Profile confirmed March 1996

ORIGINAL PERFORMANCE MEASURE SOURCE/DEVELOPER

Joint Commission

Clinical Performance

Pregnancy/Maternal Care

PERFORMANCE MEASURE PROFILE

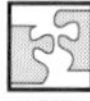 *Appropriateness*

 *Availability*

 *Continuity*

 *Effectiveness*

 *Efficiency*

 *Prevention/Early Detection*

 *Timeliness*

PERFORMANCE MEASURE

Prenatal care in first trimester.

FOCUS OF MEASURE

Prenatal care.

RATIONALE

Entry into prenatal care in the first trimester is generally believed to improve pregnancy outcome. According to the Congressional Office of Technology Assessment, women who receive better prenatal care have improved pregnancy outcomes regardless of race and socioeconomic status. The Institute of Medicine estimated that the costs of prenatal care beginning in the first trimester for all mothers reduced low birthweight by 9%. They calculated that for every one dollar spent on prenatal care, $3.38 would be saved in avoiding the medical care costs related to the treatment of low birthweight infants.

TYPE OF MEASURE

Process

NUMERATOR STATEMENT

1. As determined by hospital discharge data and ambulatory encounter data, the number of women in the denominator population who had a prenatal visit 26-44 weeks prior to delivery (or prior to estimated date of confinement [EDC], if known). Note: the numerator is calculated retroactively from time of delivery or EDC.
2. As determined in the medical record review, the number of women in the sample who had a prenatal visit 26-44 weeks prior to delivery (or prior to EDC, if known). Note: the numerator is calculated retroactively from time of delivery or EDC.
3. As determined by administrative data or in the medical record review, the number of women in the sample who had a prenatal visit 26-44 weeks prior to delivery (or prior to EDC, if known). Note: the numerator is calculated retroactively from time of delivery or EDC.

Numerator Description

Data Element(s):

A. Member ID
B. Procedure
C. Date of service

Corresponding Data Source(s):

1. Administrative data (A-C)
2. Medical record (A-C)
3. Administrative data and/or medical record (A-C)

Included Populations:

1. A woman is counted as receiving prenatal care in the first trimester, if one of the following services (noted by either a CPT-4 procedure codes or ICD-9-CM diagnosis code) is rendered 26-44 weeks prior to delivery or EDC: CPT-4 59510, 59400, 59425, or 59426 OR CPT-4 99201-99205 or 99211-99215, in conjunction with both of the following: ICD-9-CM diagnosis codes 640.0x-648.9x or 651.0x-659.9x (5th digit=3) or V22.0-V23.9 by itself; AND CPT-4 80055 or 86762 with 86900, 86901, 86105, or 86115 OR CPT-4 99201-99205 or 99211-99215, in conjunction with: internal plan code denoting complete obstetrical history with documentation of last mestrual period (LMP) or EDC.
2. A woman is counted as receiving prenatal care in the first trimester if her medical record contains evidence of a standardized method of presenting a complete obstetrical history (such as, a standardized prenatal OB form) in conjunction with rubella antibody testing and Rh/ABO blood typing within 26-44 weeks before delivery or EDC. The services may be completed during any visit during the first trimester.
3. A woman is counted as receiving prenatal care in the first trimester if either 1 or 2 is satisfied.

Excluded Populations: None

DENOMINATOR STATEMENT

1. All women who were 10-49 years of age as of the delivery date, who had a live birth(s) during the reporting period, and who were continuously enrolled for 12 months prior to delivery. Deliveries resulting in live births may be identified as women discharged with a principal or secondary diagnosis code of DRG codes 370-375. Only deliveries resulting in live births should be included. It is the plan's responsibility to document their methodology for validating live births when using DRGs; or ICD-9-CM diagnosis codes 650.xx or V codes 27.0, 27.2, 27.3, 27.5, or 27.6; or an equivalent method used by the health plan to document live births. The plan must

Continued on following page

document the method, including codes used, for validating live births. V codes may be verified by the following principal or secondary ICD-9-CM diagnosis codes 640-648.9 with a fifth digit equal to "1" or "2," or 651-656.3 with a fifth digit equal to "1" or "2," or 656.5-676.9 with a fifth digit equal to "1" or "2," or 669.5x-669.7x.

2. A random sample of 384 women members, drawn from the health plan's eligible population, 10-49 years of age as of the delivery date, who had a live birth(s) during the reporting period, and who were continuously enrolled for 12 months prior to delivery. Deliveries resulting in live births may be identified as women discharged with a principal or secondary diagnosis code of DRG codes 370-375. Only deliveries resulting in live births should be included. It is the plan's responsibility to document their methodology for validating live births when using DRGs; or ICD-9-CM diagnosis codes 650.xx; or V codes: 27.0, 27.2, 27.3, 27.5, or 27.6; or an equivalent method used by the health plan to document live births. The plan must document the method, including codes used, for validating live births. V codes may be verified by the following principal or secondary ICD-9-CM diagnosis codes 640-648.9 with a fifth digit equal to "1" or "2," or 651-656.3 with a fifth digit equal to "1" or 2," or 656.5-676.9 with a fifth digit equal to "1" or "2," or 669.5x-669.7x.

3. A random sample of 384 women members, drawn from the health plan's eligible population, 10-49 years of age as of the delivery date, who had a live birth(s) during the reporting period, and who were continuously enrolled for 12 months prior to delivery. Deliveries resulting in live births may be identified as women discharged with a principal or secondary diagnosis code of DRG codes 370-375. Only deliveries in live births should be included. It is the plan's responsibility to document their methodology for validating live births when using DRGs; or ICD-9-CM diagnosis codes 650.xx; or V codes 27.0, 27.2, 27.3, 27.5, or 27.6; or an equivalent method used by the health plan to document live births. The plan must document the method, including codes used, for validating live births. V codes may be verified by the following principal or secondary ICD-9-CM diagnosis codes 640-648.9 with a fifth digit equal to "1" or "2," or 651-656.3 with a fifth digit equal to "1" or "2," or 656.5-676.9 with a fifth digit equal to "1" or "2," or 669.5x-669.7x.

Denominator Description

Data Element(s):

A. Member ID
B. Member age (date of birth)
C. Enrollment eligibility/date
D. Payer group (for example, HMO, POS, PPO)
E. Product type (for example, commercial)
F. Delivery date or EDC
G. Delivery status (for example, live birth, stillborn)

Corresponding Data Source(s):

A-G. Administrative data

Included Populations: All women who delivered a live birth; live births that took place in a birthing center

Excluded Populations: Women whose deliveries did not result in a live birth

DOMAINS OF PERFORMANCE

Domain	
Appropriateness	Yes
Availability	Yes
Continuity	Yes
Effectiveness	Yes
Efficacy	No
Efficiency	Yes
Prevention/Early Detection	Yes
Respect and Caring	No
Safety	No
Timeliness	Yes

DELIVERY SETTINGS	Initial Settings	Applicable Settings
Health Care Network/Plan	✓	✓
Hospital		
Practitioner Office	✓	✓
Ambulatory Care Clinic		✓
Behavioral Health		
Home Care		
Nursing Home		
Subacute Care Setting		
Rehabilitation Setting		
Hospice		
Clinical Laboratory		

Continued on following page

Clinical Performance

Pregnancy/Maternal Care

Continued from previous page

Clinical Performance

Pregnancy/Maternal Care

Continued from previous page

TESTING

Reliability . . . . No
Validity . . . . No
Relevance . . . . No
Discriminatory Capability. . . . . No
Data Collection Effort . . . . Yes
Denominator Verification . . . . No

STRATIFICATION

No

RISK ADJUSTMENT

No

CURRENT DEVELOPMENT STATUS

Measure was implemented.

ADDITIONAL INFORMATION

1. Administrative data specification
2. Medical record review specification
3. Hybrid method specification

SUBMITTING ORGANIZATION

National Committee for Quality Assurance (NCQA), HEDIS 2.5
Profile confirmed March 1996

ORIGINAL PERFORMANCE MEASURE SOURCE/DEVELOPER

NCQA

PERFORMANCE MEASURE
Ambulatory surgical patient admitted or retained for complication of surgery or anesthesia.

FOCUS OF MEASURE
Provider quality and utilization; risk management outpatient diagnoses and procedures.

RATIONALE
To monitor quality of care.

TYPE OF MEASURE
Not provided

NUMERATOR STATEMENT
All patients admitted or retained unexpectedly following a complication of outpatient surgery or anesthesia event.

Numerator Description
Not provided

DENOMINATOR STATEMENT
All patients undergoing an ambulatory procedure.

Denominator Description
Not provided

DOMAINS OF PERFORMANCE
Appropriateness........................ No
Availability........................... No
Continuity............................. No
Effectiveness.......................... Yes
Efficacy............................... Yes
Efficiency............................. Yes
Prevention/Early Detection............. No
Respect and Caring..................... No
Safety................................. No
Timeliness............................. No

DELIVERY SETTINGS	Initial Settings	Applicable Settings
Health Care Network/Plan	✓	✓
Hospital	✓	✓
Practitioner Office		
Ambulatory Care Clinic	✓	✓
Behavioral Health		
Home Care		
Nursing Home		
Subacute Care Setting		
Rehabilitation Setting		
Hospice		
Clinical Laboratory		

TESTING
Not provided

STRATIFICATION
Not provided

RISK ADJUSTMENT
Not provided

CURRENT DEVELOPMENT STATUS
Measure was implemented.

ADDITIONAL INFORMATION
Not applicable

SUBMITTING ORGANIZATION
Sagamore Health Network
Profile confirmed April 1996

ORIGINAL PERFORMANCE MEASURE SOURCE/DEVELOPER
Sagamore Health Network

Clinical Performance

Procedure Complications

PERFORMANCE MEASURE PROFILE

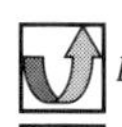 *Effectiveness*

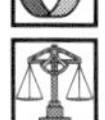 *Efficacy*

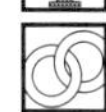 *Efficiency*

0117-00223

PERFORMANCE MEASURE

Condition specific TyPEs (Technology of Patient Experience): rheumatoid arthritis TyPE specification—rheumatoid arthritis forms 7.1–7.3.

FOCUS OF MEASURE

Evaluation of disease activity for patients with rheumatoid arthritis.

RATIONALE

To provide a data collection instrument that yields the minimum set of data elements describing the patient's experience, that supplies maximum information for the clinical management of treatment procedures and protocols, while relieving the burden of data collection on the patient as well as the practitioner.

TYPE OF MEASURE

Outcome

OTHER STATEMENT

This data collection protocol analyzes the status (patients with rheumatoid arthritis) by cross section and longitude. Variables considered most important in patient outcomes are identified, as well as characteristics necessary for making an appropriate diagnosis and evaluating disease activity.

Other Description

Data Element(s): Rheumatoid arthritis TyPE specification forms

Corresponding Data Source(s): Patient and practitioners

Included Populations: Patients 14 years of age or older who are able to use a self-administered questionnaire, and who have rheumatoid arthritis

Excluded Populations: Patients less than 14 years old and those who do not have rheumatoid arthritis

DOMAINS OF PERFORMANCE

Appropriateness....... No
Availability....... No
Continuity....... No
Effectiveness....... Yes
Efficacy....... Yes
Efficiency....... No
Prevention/Early Detection....... Yes
Respect and Caring....... No
Safety....... No
Timeliness....... No

DELIVERY SETTINGS

	Initial Settings	Applicable Settings
Health Care Network/Plan	✓	✓
Hospital		
Practitioner Office	✓	✓
Ambulatory Care Clinic	✓	✓
Behavioral Health		✓
Home Care		✓
Nursing Home		
Subacute Care Setting		
Rehabilitation Setting		✓
Hospice		
Clinical Laboratory		

TESTING

Reliability....... Yes
Validity....... Yes
Relevance....... Yes
Discriminatory Capability....... Yes
Data Collection Effort....... Yes
Denominator Verification....... No

STRATIFICATION

No

RISK ADJUSTMENT

No

CURRENT DEVELOPMENT STATUS

Measure was pilot tested and implemented.

ADDITIONAL INFORMATION

Not applicable

SUBMITTING ORGANIZATION

Health Outcomes Institute
Profile confirmed March 1996

ORIGINAL PERFORMANCE MEASURE SOURCE/DEVELOPER

Health Outcomes Institute

Health Status
Clinical Performance

Arthritis

PERFORMANCE MEASURE PROFILE

 *Effectiveness*

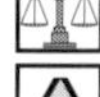 *Efficacy*

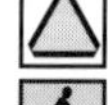 *Prevention/Early Detection*

 *Physical Functioning*

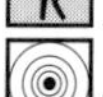 *Role Functioning–Physical*

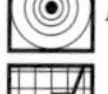 *Bodily Pain*

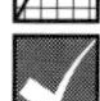 *General Health*

Reported Health Transition

0107-00117

PERFORMANCE MEASURE

Visit specific satisfaction survey.

FOCUS OF MEASURE

To assess patient satisfaction with major dimensions of care and services provided; provide overall rating of care and services provided in practice; compare patient satisfaction with the care and services provided against internally and externally derived references; identify system problems adversely affecting delivery of high quality care.

RATIONALE

To assess patient satisfaction with major dimensions of the care and services provided, provide an overall rating of the care and services provided in the practice, compare patient satisfaction with the care and services provided against internally and externally derived references, identify system problems that may adversely affect delivery of high quality patient care.

TYPE OF MEASURE

Outcome

OTHER STATEMENT

Visit specific satisfaction survey.

Other Description

Data Element(s): Visit specific satisfaction survey

Corresponding Data Source(s): Patient

Included Populations: Patients 14 years of age or older who are able to use a self-administered questionnaire, who are in a primary care setting

Excluded Populations: Patients less than 14 years of age who are not patients in a primary care setting

DOMAINS OF PERFORMANCE

Appropriateness........................ No
Availability........................... Yes
Continuity .... Yes
Effectiveness.......................... No
Efficacy .... No
Efficiency .... No
Prevention/Early Detection .... Yes
Respect and Caring .... Yes
Safety .... No
Timeliness............................. No

DELIVERY SETTINGS	Initial Settings	Applicable Settings
Health Care Network/Plan	✓	✓
Hospital		✓
Practitioner Office	✓	✓
Ambulatory Care Clinic	✓	✓
Behavioral Health		✓
Home Care	✓	✓
Nursing Home		
Subacute Care Setting		
Rehabilitation Setting	✓	✓
Hospice		
Clinical Laboratory		

TESTING

Reliability............................ Yes
Validity............................... Yes
Relevance.............................. Yes
Discriminatory Capability .... Yes
Data Collection Effort .... Yes
Denominator Verification .... No

STRATIFICATION

Yes

RISK ADJUSTMENT

Yes

CURRENT DEVELOPMENT STATUS

Measure was pilot tested and implemented.

ADDITIONAL INFORMATION

Not applicable

SUBMITTING ORGANIZATION

Health Outcomes Institute

Profile confirmed March 1996

ORIGINAL PERFORMANCE MEASURE SOURCE/DEVELOPER

Health Outcomes Institute

Satisfaction

Patient/Enrollee Satisfaction

PERFORMANCE MEASURE PROFILE

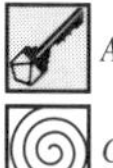
Availability

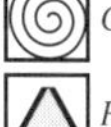
Continuity

Prevention/Early Detection

Respect and Caring

Satisfaction

Patient/Enrollee Satisfaction

PERFORMANCE MEASURE PROFILE

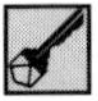 *Availability*

 *Efficiency*

 *Timeliness*

PERFORMANCE MEASURE

Member satisfaction: access/appointment wait times for serious problems and for well care visits.

FOCUS OF MEASURE

Appointment wait times.

RATIONALE

To meet patients' and members' expectations for access to meet their needs.

TYPE OF MEASURE

Outcome

NUMERATOR STATEMENT

Patients rating access to provider as very good or excellent.

Numerator Description

Data Element(s): Respondents rating very good or excellent (4/5 or 5/5) on a five-point scale

Corresponding Data Source(s): Mailed survey of members having seen particular provider for an appointment kept

Included Populations: Not applicable

Excluded Populations: None

DENOMINATOR STATEMENT

Patients seeing a particular provider for appointment kept.

Denominator Description

Data Element(s): Yearly 10% random sample of provider appointments (2.5% each quarter)

Corresponding Data Source(s): Automated visit registration system (that is, patient registration for visit, not appointments made)

Included Populations: Random sample of all patients who saw particular provider for an appointment kept

Excluded Populations: None

DOMAINS OF PERFORMANCE

Domain	
Appropriateness	No
Availability	Yes
Continuity	No
Effectiveness	No
Efficacy	No
Efficiency	Yes
Prevention/Early Detection	No
Respect and Caring	No
Safety	No
Timeliness	Yes

DELIVERY SETTINGS

DELIVERY SETTINGS	Initial Settings	Applicable Settings
Health Care Network/Plan	✓	✓
Hospital		NP
Practitioner Office	✓	✓
Ambulatory Care Clinic	✓	✓
Behavioral Health	✓	✓
Home Care		NP
Nursing Home		NP
Subacute Care Setting		NP
Rehabilitation Setting		NP
Hospice		NP
Clinical Laboratory		NP

NP = Not provided

Continued on following page

0113-00186

TESTING
Not provided

STRATIFICATION
No

RISK ADJUSTMENT
No

CURRENT DEVELOPMENT STATUS
Measure was implemented.

ADDITIONAL INFORMATION
Not applicable

SUBMITTING ORGANIZATION
Kaiser Permanente (Northern California)
Profile confirmed February 1996

ORIGINAL PERFORMANCE MEASURE SOURCE/DEVELOPER
Kaiser Permanente (Northern California)

Satisfaction

Patient/Enrollee Satisfaction

Continued from previous page

Administrative/Financial

Utilization

PERFORMANCE MEASURE PROFILE

PERFORMANCE MEASURE
Members receiving chemical dependency services: ambulatory care.

FOCUS OF MEASURE
Chemical dependency.

RATIONALE
Provide users with information to assess plan expenditures and utilization.

TYPE OF MEASURE
Process

OTHER STATEMENT
Report by gender and age cohort number of ambulatory chemical dependency services utilized during the reporting year and the percentage of members in a specific age/gender cohort utilizing ambulatory, chemical dependency care. Members receiving ambulatory chemical dependency services may be captured by using the ICD-9-CM diagnosis codes (291-292.9; 303.0-305.93; 965.0x; 965.8x; 967.xx; 968.5x; or 969.xx) in conjunction with CPT-4 procedures codes: 90801, Diagnostic Assessment; 90820, Interactive Interview Examination; 90841, MD Psychotherapy; 90842, MD Psychotherapy; 90843, MD Psychotherapy; 90844, MD Psychotherapy; 90844.22, MD Psychotherapy; 90846, Family Psychotherapy without patient; 90847, Family Psychotherapy; 90847.22, Family Psychotherapy Discretionary; 90849, Multi-family Group Therapy; 90853, Group Psychotherapy; 90855, Interactive Individual Medical Psychotherapy; 90857, Interactive Group Medical Psychotherapy; 90862, Pharmacology Management; 90870-90871, Electroconvulsive Therapy; 98900, Medical Assessment; 98902, Conference between patient and MD. Separate ambulatory services as follows: "revenue" codes: 900–903, 909–911, 914–916, 918, 919; and "type of bill" code 13x (Hospital Outpatient) or 43x (Christian Science Hospital Outpatient), where "x" equals any third digit.

Other Description
Data Element(s):

A. Member ID
B. Member age (date of birth)
C. Gender
D. Date of service
E. Procedure
F. Revenue code/type of bill code
G. Diagnosis

Corresponding Data Source(s):

A-G. Administrative data

Included Populations: Ambulatory services delivered in any setting (such as, hospital outpatient clinic, physician's office) should be counted as ambulatory services

Excluded Populations: Day/night and inpatient services; mental health

DOMAINS OF PERFORMANCE

Appropriateness	No
Availability	No
Continuity	No
Effectiveness	No
Efficacy	No
Efficiency	No
Prevention/Early Detection	No
Respect and Caring	No
Safety	No
Timeliness	No

DELIVERY SETTINGS	Initial Settings	Applicable Settings
Health Care Network/Plan	✓	✓
Hospital		
Practitioner Office	✓	✓
Ambulatory Care Clinic	✓	✓
Behavioral Health	✓	✓
Home Care		
Nursing Home		
Subacute Care Setting		
Rehabilitation Setting		
Hospice		
Clinical Laboratory		

Continued on following page

0121-00252

TESTING

Reliability . . . . No
Validity . . . . No
Relevance . . . . No
Discriminatory Capability. . . . . No
Data Collection Effort . . . . No
Denominator Verification . . . . No

STRATIFICATION

Yes

RISK ADJUSTMENT

No

CURRENT DEVELOPMENT STATUS

Measure was implemented.

ADDITIONAL INFORMATION

Not applicable

SUBMITTING ORGANIZATION

National Committee for Quality Assurance (NCQA), HEDIS 2.5
Profile confirmed March 1996

ORIGINAL PERFORMANCE MEASURE SOURCE/DEVELOPER

NCQA

Administrative/Financial

Utilization

Continued from previous page

APPENDIX B: Optimizing Teams and Teamwork

Chapter Highlights

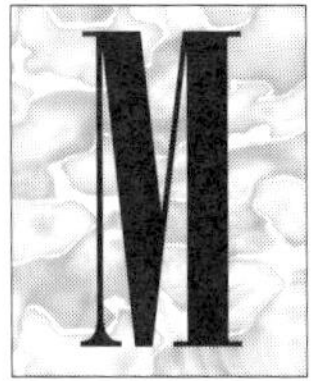

Most people have experienced the frustration of committees—their purpose is unclear, meetings ramble, one member dominates the discussion, no one speaks up, the chairperson is too dogmatic or offers no direction, turf battles dominate discussions, no one has the necessary expertise or the necessary data, everyone believes he or she has the answer but no one listens to each other, the group cannot reach consensus even about meeting dates and times, members are consistently late or absent. . . . The unhappy list seems to go on forever.

To eliminate some of these problems, eliminate the word *committee* for purposes of this discussion. *Committee* implies a permanent body with a broad, static purpose. Instead, use the word *team,* the term commonly employed for quality improvement. Teams are a vital part of behavioral health practice, including clinical teams, quality teams, and special focus teams. *Team* implies a group working together for a well-defined purpose. It also implies a group that will not be together forever, a particularly bleak and tiring aspect of some committees. Indeed, once a specific project or a series of projects is completed, a team often disbands—with a positive sense of accomplishment.

This appendix examines ground rules, team stages, and roles, and surveys some of the ingredients of a successful team. The overriding purpose of this discussion is to avoid the traps of a dysfunctional group described in the first paragraph.

Teams

Teams need structure, support, and time to grow. Do not expect a team to function at peak efficiency at the first or at every subsequent meeting. Like any group of people, the members of the improvement team must go through many stages in its life cycle. These stages include various mixtures of work and productivity.

Establishing major team tasks includes

- selecting the team;
- setting group rules;
- doing the groundwork;
- conducting team meetings and tracking outcomes; and
- completing the task.

Ground Rules: Begin at the Beginning

Setting the ground rules at the outset can help a team avoid endless distractions and detours on the road to improvement. Look at the ground rules as an opportunity to design a framework that allows the team to function smoothly. These typically include:

Decision making. The group must decide what kind of consensus or majority is needed for a decision, recognizing that decisions belong to the entire team.

Attendance. Attendance is crucial. Constant late arrivals and absences can sabotage the team's efforts. Set guidelines for attendance and hold to them.

Meeting schedule. For high attendance and steady progress, the team should agree on a regular time, day, and place for meetings. Also, the team should determine the frequency of meetings. These matters should be revisited at various times during the team's life.

Opportunity to speak. By agreeing at the outset to give all members an opportunity to contribute and to be heard with respect, the team will focus its attention on the important area of open communication.

Disagreements. The team must openly agree to disagree. It must acknowledge and accept that members will openly debate differences in viewpoint. It is fine for discussions to overflow outside the meeting room, but members should never feel that what they say in the hallway cannot be said in the meeting.

Assignments. The team should agree to complete assignments within the particular time limits so that delayed work from an individual does not delay the group.

Other rules. The team should discuss all other rules that members feel are important. These can include whether senior management staff can attend, whether pocket pagers should be checked at the door, what the break frequency is, and so forth.

Team Roles

A team should function within a framework that will provide for its mission, support its activities through various resources, furnish it with reporting channels, and give it authority. This framework, in part, takes the form of roles for team members. Fulfilling these roles is necessary if a team is to progress steadily in its efforts.

Team Leader (Facilitator)

The team leader may be established before the rest of the team forms or may be selected at the first team meeting. Even if a team leader is designated before the team forms, the role of facilitating the meetings can be taken by another team member and may be changed several times during the project, or even during a single meeting. The facilitator's role is to be objective and to move the team along.

No matter who takes the baton, the team leader/facilitator must fulfill these essential duties:

Keep the discussion moving forward within the allotted time frame. A sagging, digressing discussion can ruin forward momentum, adversely affect morale, hurt the leader's image, and put the team behind schedule. The leader should keep the discussion moving by containing digression, getting input from a variety of members, taking steps to reach consensus, introducing new topics, and ensuring that the team does not go too far beyond time limits set for each agenda item.

Pull the group together if the discussion fragments into multiple conversations. A team is not functioning as a whole when three groups are talking at once. The leader must stop such confusion quickly and, without being dictatorial, have one member speak at a time.

Encourage input from quiet members. All members have important ideas to impart; sometimes quiet members have the most interesting ideas. Perhaps they remain silent simply because their ideas seem different from everyone else's ideas. In any case, a leader can use several methods to draw out quiet members. One method is to go around the table, asking for brief comments from everyone. Another approach is to ask the quiet members directly for their ideas (for some members, this may be too threatening) or to ask these members for their ideas outside the meeting. In any case, the leader must validate the member's contribution, so that he or she—and other quiet members as well—will be more likely to contribute as the process moves on.

Prevent domination by one group member. To remedy this problem, the leader can ask for short contributions from everyone, or from specific members. The leader can also put an arbitrary time limit on comments (at the risk of seeming too domineering). Another idea is for the leader to ask all members to write short comments anonymously, distribute them randomly around the table, and read them aloud. Perhaps one of the most effective remedies is for the leader to speak privately with the member dominating the group, politely asking him or her to allow others equal time.

Check for consensus or group decisions. The leader should not try to make decisions for the group. He or she must guide the group through the sometimes difficult process of reaching a consensus decision. This may or may not be reached by a unanimous vote. Team decision making tools discussed on page 108 can be very helpful. Indeed, unanimity is rare and not necessarily desirable. Reaching consensus requires getting all members' views, building respect for various views, objectively weighing the implications of each view, and recognizing that rarely will a decision please all members.

Work with the person or group overseeing the team to report its progress. Such reports require the ability to summarize information supported by accurate records. The leader also delegates details such as keeping records and scheduling meetings, and may also coordinate any added education for members (for example, in indicator monitoring).

Recorder

As the name denotes, this member keeps a written record of meetings. He or she also can set or document agendas, compile minutes, and secure needed documents for the team. This assignment may not seem like a prize, but it is vital to efficient functioning; therefore, it should be rotated among members without considering rank in the organization.

Quality Expert

This member has special expertise in quality assessment and improvement; a project staff person may fit this role. This person should be familiar with quality improvement tools and have excellent teaching skills. If additional expertise is needed, the team may use consultants or other outside experts in statistics, engineering, market research, and so on.

Team Member

Ultimately, responsibility for a team's success rests with the members. Each member participates in discussions, performs specific assignments (such as data collection), contributes his or her expertise and creativity, and may help implement actions. Members also carry out specific roles (such as recorder or facilitator) as necessary. Although a team leader may be the most visible presence, each member must know that without his or her unique contribution, the process can falter. Quality improvement, after all, includes mutual respect and cooperation about effective communication and removal of barriers.

Team Stages

Getting Acquainted and Getting Started

Perhaps little will be done to improve the quality of health care delivery at this stage, but what takes place early in the team's life can determine how well it will function in the future. In this early stage, members become familiar with each other. Team members from diverse backgrounds may have had little direct communication in the past or may not have communicated as equals. Perhaps different constituent representatives sitting around the table harbor preconceived notions about each other, which will be tested during the getting-acquainted stage. Later in the group's life, these notions will probably be disproved.

Members will want to see how the team leader functions. Will he or she be dominant or passive? Will he or she be open to ideas from all members? Will the environment be constructive, destructive, invigorating, or stifling? Will the leader encourage all members to speak, or will he or she allow certain members to dominate discussions? Will the leader keep the group on track when it wanders? Does the leader have a hidden agenda?

In this early stage, members will often speak gingerly, testing the waters, waiting to see whether they will be able to speak their minds comfortably. Response from the leader and from other members at this tender stage will often determine the quality of later participation.

At first, the team will be unsure of its duties and goals. Members may be hopeful that improvement is possible or may be skeptical about the entire process. At this stage, members should be encouraged to introduce themselves, share ideas openly, and define and explore the task at hand. The team should know that it will not make great strides in the first several meetings; this is the time for clarifying goals and becoming comfortable as a team.

Getting Underway

A team must go through certain growing pains and developmental stages. Even when the most competent and secure person or group tackles a large project, some fear occurs. The project looks too big, too complex. The people feel they do not have the time or the skills. Answers based on experience or anecdotal evidence may be advanced and found wanting. Members may not be sure how to proceed—the first step is often the hardest to choose. Prejudices, hidden agendas, and other conflicts among team members may surface. Team members may be contentious or overly polite. Neither behavior is necessarily productive.

At this stage, teams may find the path to their goal obscure, and any spirit of optimism may wane. As in any relationship, the key is not jumping ship. If members can work through the panic and pain, the relationship becomes stronger and the members gain mutual respect. This stage can also be productive in terms of the improvement task at hand. If members initially thought a process was simple and easy to improve, this stage may bring the realization that most processes are very complex.

The earlier stages of team building may not show demonstrative progress toward improving the quality of health care delivery, but they are necessary for team growth and success. To get through this stage with the team intact, the leader needs to allow enough freedom for members to air their concerns, but should not let the group deteriorate into diatribes, war stories, or sullen silence. The leader must be especially skilled in the techniques that help groups create ideas and reach consensus. Above all, the leader must show faith in the process and must reassure the team that beyond the pain lies productivity.

Team Building

Having survived some difficulty, the group should emerge with renewed confidence and new interpersonal skills. At this point, a more cohesive group begins to form as members realize that the sum of the group can produce a better result than any individual effort. Previously competitive relationships become more cooperative, and individual agendas are adjusted to meet the group's needs. Disagreements are open and honest, and members actively listen to each other. Understanding, compromise, trust, and openness are the norm.

As a result, creative ideas begin to emerge, and members see real hope for improvement. In short, team members respect and accept each other, and they feel good about what they are doing as a team. At this stage, the leader must channel the energy into productive problem analysis and problem solving.

Team Work

The team is now comfortable about settling conflicts or disagreements; it has established and become comfortable with its criteria and rules, and has begun to demonstrate true problem-solving behavior. At this stage, the team is also becoming more knowledgeable about the issues at hand: the health care delivery network; structure, process, and outcome; indicator monitoring; and so on.

The leadership role changes at this point. If a firm hand was sometimes necessary in the previous steps, team members may now require less guidance. If a team needed motivation or reassurance before, it now may have grown beyond that need. In fact, the team may now require slowing at times.

One pitfall of this stage is regression. Any number of circumstances can move a team back to a previous stage: loss of a member, new members, an unsuccessful test, or a new directive from a steering committee or administration. The leader may need to remind the group that regression is an expected part of the process.

In addition, all members should know that the duration and intensity of these stages will vary. A team that is not progressing the way it wants should not be demoralized; rather, it should understand that lack of progression at this stage is normal, and it should look for the tools necessary to improve the team's efforts.

A Team Improvement Cycle

Once underway, improvement work with teams follows an improvement cycle. The following steps are adapted from *The Team Handbook:*

Clarify Goals

- Discuss mission statement
- Create an improvement plan

Educate and Build the Team

- Start building the team
- Set ground rules and logistics
- Discuss quality issues
- Educate team members about quality improvement tools

Investigate the Process

- Describe the process or problem
- Localize problems
- Look for root causes
- Test and refine data collection procedures

Analyze Data and Seek Solutions

- Look for patterns in the data
- Explore schematic solutions
- Develop a strategy for further improvement

Take Appropriate Action

- Look back for further investigation
- Design or redesign the product or process
- Standardize procedures
- Stabilize the process
- Monitor the results of all changes—evaluate and refine as needed
- Document progress

Establish Closure

- Evaluate the team's process
- Evaluate the project's results
- Organize files
- Update picture book format
- Make final presentation
- Recommend follow-up activities

Ingredients for a Successful Team

Some tips for creating and maintaining a successful team include the following:

- Identify team goals. Members will need to know what will be expected from the project.
- Prepare a mission statement. With a mission statement, the team will understand its purpose, limitations, expectations, authority, composition, and structure.
- Determine resources. This will help the team know what education, budget, expertise, and so forth are needed.

- Select the team leader. Through whatever process the organization chooses, a leader who is knowledgeable, interested, and skilled should be selected.
- Assign the project advisor. If the advisor is different from the leader, this person should be identified.
- Select project teams. If subteams are required, they should be small and composed of parties involved with the task at hand.
- Use agendas. Agendas will help keep meetings on track.
- Use effective discussion skills. These should include asking for clarification, listening, summarizing, minimizing digression, managing time, and testing for consensus.
- Set up a record-keeping system. Agendas, minutes, and documents are ways to track a team's work.
- Set group rules. Matters such as attendance, promptness, meeting place and time, the importance of full participation, and so on should be decided up front.

Some additional attributes found in successful teams include:

- An improvement plan that is developed to help the team determine what advice, assistance, training, materials, and other resources it may need.
- Beneficial team behaviors. All members are encouraged to use the skills and practices that make discussions and meetings effective.
- Participants who believe in and are committed to the value of working together in a spirit of cooperation.
- Team size that is appropriate for effective communication.
- Participants who understand the overall objectives of the project.
- Participants who understand individual roles and responsibilities, as well as relationships to other staff members.
- Participants who take the time to establish and clarify guidelines and procedures for a working relationship; they are committed to making plans and achieving them.
- Participants who define and agree on meaningful and measurable objectives that meet both group and personal needs; individuality and creativity are not stifled.
- Someone within the group who assumes leadership to coordinate each task or program effort.

- Participants who function well in a variety of roles (initiating, informing, summarizing, mediating, encouraging) and know when appropriate roles are needed.
- Participants who know each other. That is, they are aware of each other's resources, skills, and expertise. They know what each person can contribute to the group.
- A group that allows sufficient time for the teamwork effort.
- A group that places work first, but also allows social interaction.

Finally, here are some additional thoughts to keep in mind when working with teams:*

- Teams are about culture change and power shifts.
- Leadership must clearly articulate the new team-based culture in its vision, values, systems, and support structures.
- Successful and effective teams have sponsorship from all appropriate organization levels.
- Redefine the manager's role to include the roles of coach, counselor, educator, and mentor that are necessary in a team-based organization.
- Identify role model teams in your organization; although staff and managers may not always know specific ways to achieve teamwork, they will know them when they see them.
- Take every opportunity you can to let employees know that they are valued and that their opinions count.
- Do whatever it takes to break down barriers to physician involvement on teams; they are needed as expert sources, especially on clinical processes.
- Teams should not begin their work with a preconceived idea of the outcome—the tendency may be to focus on the wrong areas. Instead, teams should let data guide their work.
- Get more staff involved in your teams; staff generally have the most realistic picture of the process.
- Most teams go through form-storm-norm-perform phases that facilitate team building.
- Requirements for teams to be effective include:
  - Appropriate membership;
  - Clear role responsibilities;

*Phillips KM: *The Power of Health Care Teams: Strategies for Success.* Oakbrook Terrace, IL: Joint Commission on Accreditation of Healthcare Organizations, 1997.

- Efficient operating processes;
- Clear charter and goals;
- Appropriate project scope for the membership, time, costs, and other constraints;
- Willingness to do work outside team meetings;
- Clear ground rules to facilitate productive meetings; and
- Team and CQI tools to facilitate the team's ability to generate and analyze data.

References

Phillips KM: *The Power of Health Care Teams: Strategies for Success.* Oakbrook Terrace, IL: Joint Commission on Accreditation of Healthcare Organizations, 1997.

Scholtes PR. *The Team Handbook: How to Use Teams to Improve Quality.* Madison, WI: Joiner Associates, Inc, 1989.

Teamwork in Cooperative Extension Programs. Madison, WI: University of Wisconsin, 1980.

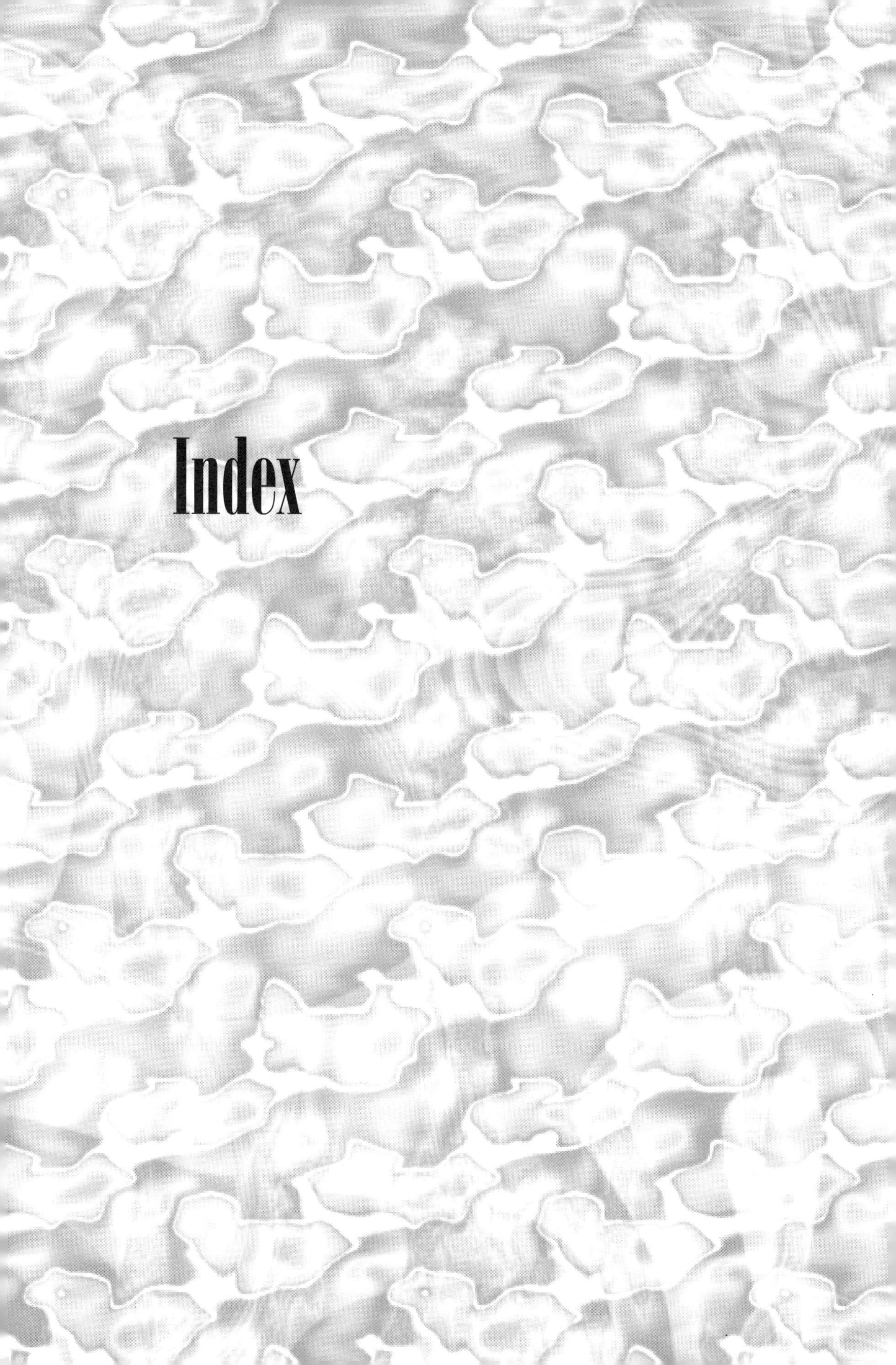

Index

f = figure
n = note
t = table